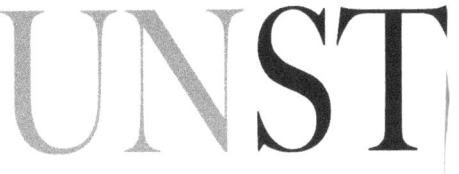

UNST

steven orenstein, ph.d.

outskirts
press

Table of Contents

1

The Beginning

AT A YOUNG age, I made a momentous decision. I was going to become a clinical psychologist. All of 15, and I knew exactly what I wanted to do.

My friends couldn't understand at all. Like me, they had outgrown dreams of being the next Mickey Mantle, the fastest gun in the west, or president of the United States. They wanted to be rock 'n roll stars, like most kids of my generation. They didn't even know what a psychologist was and had certainly never been to see one.

My parents, on the other hand, understood very well. They knew that my interest in psychology was genuine and had grown out of my own very real experience. They had been taking me to see therapists—psychiatrists, psychoanalysts, psychologists, group therapists—since I was 6 or 7 years old. The first was Dr. Shildkraut who had, in an earlier incarnation, been the obstetrician who had delivered me. Dr. Green, a very formal and stiff psychiatrist, who had tried to convince my parents to put me in the hospital or, at the very least, get me on psychiatric medications, was the last. In between, there was the psychoanalyst who fell asleep in the middle of a session, the psychiatrist who played dominos with me, and the scary, shaven-headed, mendacious Dr. Stein. They knew that none of them had had a major impact on things. I was still the same moody, precocious, angry, rebellious little snot I'd always been. But there were really no better options for a kid whose academic potential was surpassed only by his contempt for authority and convention. And I think that whenever those therapists' bills came due, my parents could take some solace in the idea that, while nothing much seemed to have changed, their son was, at least, not getting any worse. They could also see that, while I often resented their dragging me to the doctor's on Thursday afternoons, I was developing an interest in something that might lead to much better things.

What my parents didn't understand so well, but what had, finally, convinced me of my career path, was that, in the late 1960s, early 1970s, psychology was just about the coolest thing this side of the Rolling Stones. The "space age" had come upon us in the late 1950s, and the cultural interest in the exploration of outer space had been accompanied by a smaller, but similar explosion of interest in the exploration of inner space. The books, art, films, and conversations of the time had begun to reflect a prosperous, optimistic society, but also one, perhaps, whose material successes had left it uneasy and unfulfilled. People began to get interested in psychotherapy like never before. It was no longer just for the seriously ill in psychiatric hospitals or a tiny elite of well-heeled intellectuals and movie stars. Otherwise healthy, productive, successful people were getting interested in understanding themselves—their feelings and motivations—and in getting more out of their lives. Troubled people started to show a greater willingness to seek therapy as the stigma of "being in analysis" began to fade. And psychotherapy was no longer the exclusive purview of psychiatry and psychoanalysis. In fact, the most creative work in psychotherapy was being done by psychologists, who were not bound to medical orthodoxy and who had been strongly influenced by the so-called "human potential movement."

Part of the attraction that so many began to feel towards psychology in this period of time may be that it appealed to a kind of restlessness that, in previous generations, would have been interpreted as spiritual yearning. People who were troubled, but not ill, stirred by the adventurous spirit of the time, began to seek in psychotherapy some sense of deeper meaning in their lives or, maybe, a greater sense of spiritual community, one based in insight and the shared experience of emotional nakedness. Some sought these same ends by pursuing exotic Eastern religions. Some ingested psilocybin mushrooms. Some did all three. During the affluent, but chaotic, 1960s, there were many people who weren't necessarily on the verge of a breakdown but who were very much looking for a breakthrough, an answer to some deep existential dilemma or a glimpse of some greater possibility in their lives.

Psychologists took their place among the leaders, *les agents provocateurs*, of a small, but significant movement of hip, sophisticated, inner-directed, consciousness-expanding psychonauts. Psychology was pushing the envelope of human behavior, questioning social mores, liberating repressed sexual impulses, challenging complacency, finding new meanings in ancient tradition and mythology, getting the world excited about the unlimited potentials within each one of us.

I couldn't wait to be a part of it.

Sigmund Freud, though he remained a towering figure, was not central to this new humanistic, experiential, transpersonal movement. The genius of Freud's work was undeniable, but he represented a different era in western culture, one in which "liberation of the vastness of human potential" was inconceivable. His was work which helped us to understand our motivations like no other that had come before it, but which was, in the end, fatalistic. He saw the great work of psychoanalysis as something which would, when all was said and done, help make what was essentially unlivable, livable. This was hardly compatible with the idea of unlimited human potential which had begun to flourish at this time. And the women's movement, which also had begun to grow during the tumultuous late 1960s/early 1970s era, had raised important questions about Freud's treatment of women and, especially, women's sexuality.

The gurus of this new movement in psychotherapy included many who had previously been outliers, men whose work and ideas had been, in its time, deemed too strange, unconventional, outrageous. Carl Jung, whose ideas about the "collective unconscious" wound up providing a foundation for much of the psychospiritual work that began in the 1960s and continues through to this day, was a major influence. Fritz Perls, commonly known (though not totally accurately) as the founder of Gestalt therapy, was a giant in psychotherapy of the era, for his dynamic, creative techniques, his emphasis on the intensive "encounter" as a vehicle for personal growth, and his knack for coining a quotable phrase (who cannot remember that nearly ubiquitous poster with the poem that began with the words "I am not in this world to meet your expectations, and you are not in this world to meet my expectations..."?).

Wilhelm Reich, probably the least studied and understood of all, might have been among the most influential. A student of Freud who went on to make extraordinary discoveries about the mind-body relationship and the influence of energetic forces on human consciousness and behavior, Reich's persecution by the US government in the 1950s helped make him an iconic, heroic figure to many who saw their work in the human potential movement as radical and revolutionary.

The influence of drugs cannot be discounted. Psychedelic drugs, particularly LSD and marijuana, were major players in the development of this emerging psychological movement. While none of the old "masters" like Perls, Jung, Reich were associated with the use of drugs, the use of drugs by psychologists in the 1960s and early 1970s was widespread. Psychedelics were seen as keys to unlocking hidden human potentials and insights gathered in the course of drug experiences were often profound and generative. Much experimentation was done to test the therapeutic potential of psychedelic drugs and there is hardly a major thinker of the 1960s who hasn't credited his use of such substances as an important influence on his work and ideas. It may be worth noting that two of the most well-known, influential, some might even say notorious, figures of the era, Timothy Leary and Richard Alpert (Ram Dass), were PhD psychologists and members of the Harvard faculty.

The human potential movement had become so powerful by the early 1970s that the training of clinical psychologists had begun to transform in response. In earlier times, a PhD program in psychology was heavily tilted in the direction of research. Clinical psychologists were, generally, trained at major universities to be skilled researchers and statisticians. They learned to develop and administer intelligence and personality tests. If they weren't spending all of their time in academic settings, teaching and doing research, they played "second fiddle" to psychiatrists, who, up until the early 1970s, or so, provided virtually all of the psychotherapy done in America.

With psychology changing and its primary offspring—psychotherapy—emerging as a significant social phenomenon, graduate programs began to address the need for training that was done with the independent, psychotherapy-oriented clinical psychologist in mind. "Professional" schools began to emerge which provided students an opportunity to study psychology as an academic and research discipline, but also, and most importantly, to study psychotherapy. Professional schools recognized that what was exciting to young people looking to enter the field of psychology in 1975, or so, was not academic research with rats running through mazes in a laboratory, it was the opportunity to become a psychotherapist, to become a vital cog in that ever-expanding wheel of human potential.

I remember being very excited to begin my training as a clinical psychologist. Having rejected the opportunity to attend a prestigious, but conservative, training program at a large east coast university, I headed off to California full of enthusiasm. The west coast was, after all, on the leading edge of American culture at that time, and this was reflected in the field of psychology as much as anything else. East coast psychology was more staid and traditional. Freud's ideas still reigned supreme. But on the west coast, there was Gestalt therapy, and bodywork, and intensive weekend encounter groups, and Esalen, and primal therapy, and Bioenergetics, and Rolfing, and, well, yes, a lot of really nice weather and pretty girls on the beach!

In fact, my move to the west coast and into professional school training was the right one. I wound up having an extraordinary experience in graduate school, with a lot of bright, energetic, creative students around me and professors who embodied the adventurous, expansive spirit of the time. I was given a terrific opportunity to get exposed to, and learn from, some of the greatest teachers, wizards, and wise ones of the era: Stan Grof, the brilliant Czechoslovakian physician whose work with LSD and terminal cancer patients in the early 1960s foreshadowed his development of holotropic breathwork years later. Chris Downing, who could speak about Freud as if she'd just finished having lunch with him at a Viennese

café. Erv and Miriam Polster, who brought a gentle artful-
ness to Gestalt therapy. Bob Resnick, who wasn't gentle, but
whose clarity and courage had gotten me interested in Gestalt
in the first place. Carl Rogers, founder of the Center for the
Studies of the Person, whose name was synonymous with "client centered therapy." Milton Trager, physician and healer,
who'd developed an extraordinary system of bodywork useful for everything from anxiety to muscular dystrophy. Etc. etc.
Psychology graduate school in California in the 1970s was a
veritable Coney Island of transformational, mind-expanding,
genre busting, paradigm-shifting roller-coaster rides.

One of the most powerful experiences I had was with
Rolfing. Not formally associated with psychology in any
way, or even with claims to be a mind-altering kind of experience, Rolfing, or structural integration, as it had originally
been called, was the brainchild of a physicist by the name
of Ida Rolf. The whole idea behind the massage-like technique that came to bear her name was that the human
body developed misalignments in its structure as a result
of the effects of gravity, trauma, and poor body mechan-
ics. Rolfing had, as its goal, the re-alignment of the body
around its natural center of gravity. Ed Maupin, to whom
I'd gone to "get Rolfed," was a psychologist who had been
one of Ida Rolf's original group of west coast trainees, highly skilled, and was an interesting, provocative, somewhat
iconoclastic figure who'd years before left behind a position
as a medical psychologist to pursue his interest in meditation, spirituality, and body work.

What made Rolfing such a powerful experience for me was that it absolutely convinced me of the mind-body connection. While in the midst of my seventh session, during which Ed was working away at the deep muscle tensions around my jaw, his hands in my mouth, I had a terrifying vision that I'll never forget. Suddenly, as I lay there on the table, feeling a lot of pressured, burning sensation in my mouth, I opened my eyes and saw, clear as day, a man standing over me, threatening to attack me with what appeared to be two sharp metal instruments. He was wearing a bright light on a band around his head, as if he were a miner or, perhaps, a surgeon. Fearing for my life, I raised my arms up, hands protecting my face, and shouted as loudly as I could, "Go away. Get out of here. Leave me alone." Then, just as suddenly as it had appeared, the monstrous vision faded away. Ed was consoling, but couldn't help me to understand what had happened, what the origin was of this vision that had scared the bejeesus out of me.

I was convinced that I had re-experienced some kind of childhood trauma, but I had no idea what it might have been, as I had no memory of ever having been through something like that. So, I did what every good Jewish boy does when he needs some help. . . I called my mother. At first, my mother had no more of an idea what this experience might have been about than I. But, we kept talking, and, eventually, she remembered that, when I was about 4 or 5 years old, in the middle of getting my tonsils removed, there'd been a moment when I'd awakened from the anesthesia. As soon as my mother said this, in that very instant, I knew. The pain and fear of that moment of consciousness 20 years before, had, somehow, been locked away in the tight tissues of my jaw. Through the process of getting Rolfed, those deep tensions were released and, with the physical expansion and the rush of energy that got discharged, I was flooded with an eidetic image as compelling as the actual experience had been. And hours later, I wasn't scared or confused, just incredibly excited to have discovered through my own experience that the connections between mind and body that I'd been hearing about and reading about for years were as real as the nose on my face.

The work of Wilhelm Reich excited me the most. His work seemed almost dangerous, like it was something that you couldn't shake, or spill, or even approach too quickly without risking major injury. Kind of like nitroglycerine. Or kryptonite. Reich's work had, for many years, been relegated to the outer fringes of psychology and, for a twenty-year period after Reich's death in 1956—he died in a federal prison cell, having been convicted with the scantest evidence of violating a government injunction—there were very few people who were even willing to talk about Reich in formal academic or professional circles. Fortunately, by the late 1970s in California, that had begun to change, and I was able to begin to indulge my interest in the work of this peculiar, radical genius.

I'd first encountered Reich as a high school student. On an otherwise uneventful Saturday afternoon, when I was about 15 years old, I'd wandered into a used bookshop and Reich's "Function of the Orgasm" seemed to jump off the shelf at me. Scooping it up like I would have an errant issue of Playboy, I tore into the book enthusiastically, hoping to find it sexy and alluring. However, within a few moments, I discovered that it was anything but that. It was dry, scientific, not erotic in the least. But the ideas within it seemed so fascinating, so incredible, so mind-bending that reading the book had the same effect, in the end, of a powerful drug experience. My consciousness was forever changed.

Reich wrote about a lifeforce, a biological energy that ran through all living things. While this wasn't really too much different from what had been suggested over hundreds and hundreds of years of mystical tradition, Reich brought a scientific perspective to his work that you couldn't find anywhere else. Many others had spoken of prana, or ch'i, or élan vital but never before had anyone taken a disciplined scientific approach to the question.

Reich posited that there is a biological energy that underlies all life processes, that we experience the movement of this energy through our bodies as feeling, and that the efforts we make to hold back our feelings result in chronic musculoskeletal tensions, neuroses, and physical illness. The orgasm, Reich believed, served the necessary biological function of discharging all of the excess energy from the body, thereby resolving tension and restoring energetic balance. He called this energy "orgone" and spent the better part of thirty years researching, writing about, and developing techniques and devices to use orgone for therapeutic purposes.

Having consumed heartily from this great stewpot of Freud, Jung, and Reich, Gestalt and bioenergetics, Rolfing, Arica, rebirthing, and just about everything else academic, experiential, chemical, spiritual, sexual, and epistemological that graduate school—and California—had to offer, PhD in hand, I entered the world of professional psychology and psychotherapy with enormous enthusiasm and optimism. It was 1980 and every-thing seemed possible. With lots of energy and, admittedly, plenty of ego, I was set to do my part to change the world.

Psychology was the coolest thing going, and I was on its cutting edge. The human potential movement was going to be bigger than ever. We were going to supplant the psychia-trists and revolutionize healthcare, teach people new ways of creating peace and social harmony, liberate sexual energies, re-make the corporate world, and create a psychologically-minded culture all around. We were going to help people heal. The world was my oyster and my degree the sword with which I'd harvest the pearl.

But somewhere along the way, things began to change. The revolution in consciousness that so many of us foresaw in the 1970s gave way to something much more constricted. To be-gin with, psychology by the mid-1980s was no longer outside the mainstream of American life and the American healthcare system, as it had been. People were going to see psychologists. Health insurance companies were starting to pay for psycho-logical services. While there were, and, perhaps, always will be, people who continued to view psychotherapy as some-thing only for "nutcases," more and more people had come to accept psychologists as legitimate healthcare providers, much the same as they saw dentists, podiatrists, optometrists, chi-ropractors. But the human potential movement, and many of the psychologists doing more progressive work, began to get swallowed up, co-opted by what I think of as an emerging *pharmacomedinsurance* complex.

Many of us young, idealistic therapists found ourselves getting married, becoming parents, getting focused more on making money than on making waves, more on surviving in a competitive professional atmosphere than on transforming the atmosphere itself. We became more conservative, as therapists, if not as people. And many of the great elders of the human potential movement had died. Perls was gone. So was Carl Rogers, along with many others. The passing of a movement's most inspirational figures called out for a new generation of charismatic leaders and pioneers to take their place. But none really emerged.

The more conservative elements of the healthcare system weren't sitting idly by, either. Insurance companies saw what had been going on, and they certainly didn't want to pay for their subscribers' personal growth needs, even if a lack of personal growth was underlying their depression, anxiety, or persistent back pain, even if such psychotherapy could help to limit their subscribers' future use of medical services! Psychiatrists were threatened by psychologists, whose training in psychotherapy, and in the kind of outpatient therapy that most people sought, was usually far more extensive than their own. The mildly disturbed but not seriously ill, the anxious but not crazy, the unhappy but not severely depressed, the neglected wife or restless husband, the worried parent—the vast majority of people with a need for or interest in psychotherapy—weren't going to see psychiatrists.

Pharmaceutical companies were in business to make money, and therapeutic techniques which obviated, or, at least, reduced the need for, medications cut into their bottom line. The collusion between the medical profession, the health insurance industry, and the pharmaceutical industry, the pharmacomedinsurance complex, was inevitable, and really grew in power through the 1980s. It has resulted in a tremendous increase in the prescription of psychiatric medications, demands by insurance companies that patients be given psychiatric medications, and has helped to ensure not that people would have access to the best possible therapy for their health needs, but that the pharmaceutical industry would continue to make gigantic profits, the health insurance industry would continue to make gigantic profits, and the medical profession—wary not just of psychologists but the whole world of "alternative healing"—would remain "top dog."

Moreover, we were moving into generally more conservative times, socially and politically. Why our society goes through historic periods of expansion, then contraction, of progressivism, then conservatism, I don't really know. But I do know that it's true. Chart the entire course of human civilization on a graph and you'd see that we go through periods of relative expansion and relative contraction, periods when we welcome novelty and change and other periods when we resist those very things. The particular spirit of the time, the zeitgeist, gets reflected in the sociopolitical events of the time.

The open, expansive spirit of the 1960s and 1970s was well reflected in the psychology of the time. Gestalt therapy was all about growth and change, and a willingness to venture into the unknown. The 1980s and 1990s, on the other hand, brought us managed care, a zillion new pharmaceuticals for everything from "social anxiety disorder" to "adult attention deficit disorder," and more people being hospitalized on psychiatric wards than ever before.

Psychology now is very unlike the profession that I'd entered into with such enthusiasm thirty-five years ago. The psychology of today is, for the most part, as conservative as society as a whole. Many psychologists have come to de-value much of what went on in the recent past. Little Gestalt therapy goes on anymore. Very little training in bioenergetics, or in any of the so-called "depth psychology" methods, goes on any more. Fewer and fewer graduate programs teach the work of the great masters in any detail. You'd be hard pressed to find in a typical graduate program these days much discussion or research on the work of Freud, or Perls, or Jung, or, heaven forbid, the notorious Wilhelm Reich. What this has meant is that most psychologists are no longer being trained to do the kind of characterological work—therapy focused on uncovering deep underlying patterns of thought and behavior rather than on short-term symptom-removal—that was central to the growth-oriented psychotherapies.

One of the big reasons for this, I think, is that many, if not most, of my contemporaries, and most psychologists who have done their training in more recent times, have sought acceptance as "doctors" by insurance carriers and the general public. The money, the power, the prestige, of being a "doctor" in American society can be very alluring. And it hasn't been all a bad thing, either. The efforts that psychologists in America have made over the past 25 years to be seen as legitimate healthcare providers has helped secure a place for psychology in the health care system. That has been, on the whole, good for the profession, or, at least, for its economic well-being. But I wonder, sometimes, if, in its search for legitimacy, psychology has sold its humanistic soul.

After all, what is it that doctors do? They treat illness. They don't help people prevent health problems. They don't assist people with their personal growth needs, their sense of community, their quality of life, or their vitality. They don't help them explore the depths of the unconscious. They don't help them improve their relationships or develop better ways of dealing with their feelings. They're don't really provide healthcare. They treat illness.

Certainly, there are many psychologists for whom depth psychotherapy and the values embodied in the human potential movement continue to be vital. But there are, on the other hand, many for whom acceptance as a "bonafide member of the healthcare profession" is more important. And, if one wants to be so accepted, if one wants to be "a doctor" in American society, to participate in the pharmacomedinsurance complex, whether you are trained as a physician, or as a psychologist, or as a chiropractor, or whatever, you must agree to treat illness. Or, perhaps even more accurately, you must agree to treat the symptoms of an illness, and not necessarily its cause. Insurance companies want to see that the rash has cleared up, that the fibromyalgic patient is now stable on her medication, that the low back pain responded well to the analgesic, that the person suffering an anxiety disorder is now able to sleep well five nights per week, rather than two. Even if, by virtue of your training and experience, you know some things about how to stay well, improve quality of life, or enhance personal relationships, and you choose to pass that on to your clients, it's not something for which insurance companies reimburse. Health insurance does not cover health, or things that promote wellness; it covers illness. Health insurance does not cover the cost of a massage, or yoga, or meditation, or stress management, or personal growth-oriented psychotherapy. It only covers you when you're sick. If you're a psychologist who wants to participate in the system, you find illness in your patients, and you treat its symptoms.

None of this is to say that the treatment of bonafide mental illness is a waste of time. Many millions of people in our society suffer from debilitating anxiety, depression, post-traumatic syndromes, eating disorders, and other psychological disease and I think it is a wonderful thing that we now have many good psychotherapeutic techniques, as well as psychiatric medications, to help these people feel better. Certainly, everyone has benefited, as well, from the significant advances made in the pharmacological treatment of severe mental illness like schizophrenia and bi-polar disorder. It is just a terrible shame that psychology seems to have forgotten the role it used to play so prominently not only in the expansion of human potential, but in emphasizing the importance of getting down to the roots of a problem so that it can be healed for all time. This is one of the main lessons we took away from Freud: to heal a problem you've got to tear it out by its roots, not simply put a band-aid on it and pronounce it cured.

On balance, it is surely a good thing that we have techniques of short-term psychotherapy to help reduce anxiety and other common problems. I support all efforts to reduce human suffering. But is it also a good thing to have abandoned efforts to ferret out the root causes of such problems and resolve them at their core?

We have, as a culture, become so oriented towards symptom-removal, towards short-term results, towards satisfying the demands of insurance carriers and managed care companies to keep treatment "brief" that many health problems that could possibly get resolved for good don't really get resolved at all. Too little attention gets paid to the root causes of problems, without which there can be no real understanding. Without understanding there can be no learning. Without learning there can be no growth, and without growth there can be no real healing. Healing is always a mind-body experience.

With all we know about the mind-body connection and nutrition and exercise physiology and all the other dimensions of health and wellness, our American society ought to be healthier than it has ever been before. In fact, we're worse off. Our immune systems are weaker, we're more violent, we're more overweight, we're more depressed, eating disorders and sleep disorders are epidemic, we're more miserable at home and at work, and our marriages are falling apart at an unprecedented rate. We're taking more and more medications every year for illnesses that never even existed before and failing to appreciate that many of these health problems and social ills share a common root in our troubled, unexamined inner lives.

Helping to heal the inner lives of people was the main focus of psychology and psychotherapy for most of its history. It is what the great work of Freud and Jung was all about. But that focus seems to have shifted. Psychologists have become part of the system and psychology is no longer "cool," no longer "cutting edge" and no longer challenging the status quo. In an age when getting well and staying healthy and enhancing quality of life has probably never been more on peoples' minds, never has occupied so much of our public dialogue, psychology, which could be contributing so much, has had very little to say apart from offering what are now formulaic prescriptions for "stress management." The deep work of personal transformation, of inner healing, of expanding consciousness and opening up human potentials continues, but very little of it has to do with psychology and psychologists any longer.

This book represents my effort to change that. Unstuck is the result of my thirty-five plus years on the leading edge of psychology and my ongoing interest in the mind-body connection, human potential, health, and wellness. Unstuck is a guide to re-framing life experiences and provides a path to greater balance and aliveness. It offers a new perspective on the nature of personal growth and a greater vision of the potential for psychology to help people heal and truly transform their lives.

2

The Roots of Suffering

BACK WHEN I was in graduate school, all of us students got together regularly in small groups to discuss our clients. Many of the meetings were mandatory "supervision sessions" when an older, established psychologist would critique our work and offer perspective on matters of diagnosis and treatment. More often, it was just us kids, getting together later on in the evenings over a beer or a joint to share our passions, our insecurities, and our intense, yearning questions about what was really going on inside the troubled people who were coming to us for help.

Our clients were of all kinds. Different races, sizes, color, background, and "presenting problem." People showed up with anxiety, depression, problems with their children, their mothers, their fathers, their teachers, their bosses. Problems sleeping, problems with alcohol, problems with sex, problems with money. Problems with themselves. A nice general cross-section of the American public. And no matter the reason for their being in therapy, the most common thing you'd hear about a client in those many discussions we'd have was that he, or she, was, in some way, "stuck."

"Stuck" in an unhappy relationship. "Stuck" in a miserable job. "Stuck" at home. "Stuck" in a bad situation. "Stuck" with all their anger and frustration. Just about everyone with any kind of psychological problem was, in one way or another, stuck.

"Stuck" is, of course, not a clinical term. Never was and probably never will be. You won't find it anywhere in the formal Diagnostic and Statistical Manual. No psychologist or psychiatrist advertises that he specializes in treating "problems of being stuck." No health insurance carrier would process a claim form which described the patient's condition as "stuck." No pharmaceutical company sells a pill to "help alleviate the symptoms of stuckness" (although I'm sure they would if they could). But doesn't "stuck" describe so well what it really feels like to be suffering?

"I just can't seem to get out of bed."

"I feel trapped in this loveless relationship."

"Nothing I do seems to make a difference."

"I keep going around in circles."

"I'm so stressed out."

"Why do I keep making the same mistake over and over again?"

"Every night, it's the same old thing."

Aren't these all just different ways of saying, "I'm stuck?" Stuck in my own muck. Stuck in some old pattern that I just can't seem to break?

The reason why "stuck" is such an apt way of describing this kind of common human suffering is more interesting than might first appear. It's simplicity and colloquialism might make it seem too mundane a term to use. After all, "stuck" is a word we use to describe a plumbing problem or old chewing gum on the bottom of your shoe. "Stuck" means "can't move." Wouldn't words like "disorder" or "conflict" be more fitting? What about calling it "illness?" Isn't that what we usually do or, at the very least, what the insurance companies and pharmaceutical companies compel us to do?

No. In actuality, "stuck" is the perfect word to describe most ordinary human suffering precisely because it means "can't move."

Movement is essential to life.

The one thing that distinguishes more than any other what is "living" from what is "non-living" is movement. Living things move. Living things pulsate. Living things contract and expand. Non-living things don't. Living things are never completely still. Even when in a state of total rest, a person—any living being—is moving inside. Life moves through a living person even if that person is in a coma. The heart beats. The lungs expand and contract. Blood circulates. The basal electrical rhythms of the body potentiate a ceaseless cascade of inflows and outflows, diffusions, penetrations, charging and discharging. Movement is our natural state of being. Being "stuck" is unnatural and life-diminishing. Being "stuck" is like being non-living. To be stuck is to suffer.

One question you might be asking yourself at this point is, "OK. On a physical level, at the level of flesh and blood and muscle and breath, I can understand how being stuck relates to suffering and ill health. Clots and prolapses and clogs and any and all kinds of blockages in the body obviously cause pain, dysfunction, disease, and death. But what does movement have to do with the mind, with psychology, with human potential and personal growth?"

In a word: everything.

One of the most important lessons I learned from years of studying, then practicing, the work of Wilhelm Reich is that there is a lifeforce, an elan vital, a "subtle energy" that pervades our living world. What Reich called "orgone" is what the Hindus call "prana," what the acupuncturists call " ch'i," what Nikola Tesla referred to as "ether." On a physical plane, the flow of the lifeforce through the blood and tissues of our bodies enhances the microcurrents of electricity that we know are indispensable to the functioning of the heart, nervous system, and other biochemical and bio-mechanical processes essential to life. Those microcurrents of electricity underlie all of the rhythmic pulsations of the body such as the constant, repetitive "lub-dup, lub-dup" of the heart. On the non-physical plane, the lifeforce is manifest as consciousness, vitality, thought, and feeling and underlies the rhythmic pulsations of the inner life: contact and withdrawal, expansion and contraction of awareness, receptivity and resistance.

Movement is no less fundamental to our minds than it is to our bodies. The physical aspect of who we are (body) and the non-physical aspect of who we are (mind) both require movement to maximize health, wellness, and a sense of being alive. Movement in the body can be viewed, and measured, in terms of pulsation: heart beats, peristaltic action, respiration. Disorder, deficits, or hyper-activity are all signs of problems, of disease. Movement in the mind can be viewed, and measured, in terms of behavior: satisfaction of psychological needs, expression of emotion, acquisition of new learning. Minds must be able to expand and contract, to receive as well as resist, just as bodies must be able to take in air and then let it out. Being stuck in the body is associated with pain and illness, lack of energy, vitality, and pleasure; so is being stuck in the mind. An arterial blockage is often associated with a heart attack or stroke. A mental blockage ("I'm stuck") is, likewise, often associated with depression and life feeling dull, repetitive, and dreary.

And sometimes, because of the multidimensional reality in which we live, the "physical block" helps to make us feel depressed and the "mental block" raises our blood pressure. We don't exist as just bodies, or as just minds, after all. We are at least both of those things. Each aspect of who we are supports, reflects, and interacts with every other aspect. Being "stuck" isn't just a metaphor for feelings of frustration. It is a statement about our very existence. When we feel compelled to say, "I've got to get something off my chest," chances are we're not kidding.

The entire living universe is interconnected. Quantum physics has been telling us that for decades, now. Spiritual masters have been teaching that for thousands of years. Of course, the mind and body are connected. If you don't believe me, go get Rolfed!!

Lack of movement in the body is going to be reflected in some kind of mental stasis and being stuck in the mind is going to be reflected in some kind of physical stasis. Likewise, movement in one dimension will find its positive complement in the other. The mind/body relationship is constant and inevitable.

Try this simple exercise: Move your body into an uncomfortable position. Clench your jaw or scrunch up your shoulders. Twist a little too far this way, or that. Try to create some serious muscular tension for a moment. And now, as you hold this contracted and uncomfortable position..........think a pleasant thought.

What you probably found is that it's tough to do. When we're uncomfortable physically—tense or in pain—it's almost as if we lose access to positive thoughts and feelings. When we're uncomfortable in our minds, we can't feel pleasure or peace in our bodies, either. If the mental discomfort is bad enough, or chronic, we don't just lose access to good feeling in our bodies, we actually start to feel bad physically as well as mentally. Like when "stress" makes us feel we're "carrying the weight of the world on our shoulders" or when anger gives us a headache or when our revulsion at someone else's bad behavior makes us feel sick to our stomachs.

Being stuck isn't the same thing as having habits, rituals, or fixed ways of doing things. Habits can be signs of being stuck, but, more often, consistency and regularity are important in life. Most people feel best when they sleep and eat at regular times. Millions of people find that daily rituals of prayer, yoga, meditation, or mindful walking at certain times of the day helps bring them peace. Thousands of years of human experience have taught us that schedules and routines are good, even necessary, to help us feel organized, get our work done, sleep well, and maintain our energy. We're all "creatures of habit," to some extent. Anything we do that helps us feel good, function well, get our needs satisfied, helps give us a sense of purpose is a good thing.

On the other hand, if what we're doing isn't serving us, doesn't help to fulfill a sense of purpose, or bring us joy or peace and the reason why we're continuing to do it doesn't really make any sense, it's a sign of us being stuck and is a cause of suffering. This is a phenomenon which might apply to all kinds of choices we make: how and what we eat, how we deal with our feelings, how we go about our work and treat other people.

Lifeforce moves through us like electrons through a Tesla coil. And like that coil, we transform that subtle energy into something more powerful: human vitality as it is expressed in mind and body.

Or, we don't.

Sometimes we function less like a powerful transformer than as a giant capacitor, holding onto, storing energy which may, or may not, ever get utilized in a positive way. Can you imagine a crazed squirrel, storing nut after nut after nut in his tree home, but never eating any of the nuts? What would happen to his home?

The Chinese have understood for thousands of years that physical illness is, at least in part, a function of a disturbance in the movement of subtle energy through the body, an imbalance. Acupuncture meridians provide a picture of this movement and a map which Doctors of Chinese Medicine use to help them restore a healthy, balanced flow of ch'i.

What I'm suggesting here is that thought, and behavior represent manifestations of ch'i, also. In our minds, with our minds, we channel energy into the creation of thought and behavior. Thought and behavior are the expression of the lifeforce in the non-physical realm of human existence.

Everything is energy. Everything in this universe, everything we think of as "real," begins with energy. In fact, your friendly neighborhood quantum physicist (you do have one, don't you?) would tell you that even the things we think of as "physical," like a guitar string, a pizza, a chair, or a human body, aren't really solid objects at all, that empty space isn't really empty, and that everything in the living universe is in a constant cosmic energetic dance with every other thing.

In health, the human body transforms the subtle lifeforce

into glorious pulsation. The heart beats in a perfect natural rhythm. The lungs pump freely. Muscles contract and expand without struggle. We ingest, digest, and excrete without effort. We enjoy sexuality and the pleasures of our senses. We feel energized and fully alive.

In health, the human mind transforms the subtle lifeforce into a full range of thought and creative, purposeful, loving behavior.

In health, we are balanced and at peace. In health, we are unstuck.

To the extent that we are energetically balanced, that is to say that lifeforce enters, moves through us, is transformed effectively and discharged freely, we are unstuck. To the extent that this natural process is impeded or distorted, we're stuck.

Two basic energetic problems can develop: overcharge or undercharge. Think of it as "too much voltage" or "not enough voltage." Both are associated with tension; when chronic, both come to be associated with dysfunction, deterioration, and disease. Run 240 volts through a 120 volt appliance and the appliance turns on, spins out of control, then burns out, its internal wiring decimated by more power than it's designed to handle. On the other hand, try running an appliance rated at 240 volts on just 120 volts of power and the performance of the appliance will be seriously degraded—if it runs at all.

Being overcharged means that a person is containing, holding onto too much energy, not letting it move through and transform into healthy pulsation and/or life-affirming behavior.

On the physical plane, this manifests as musculoskeletal rigidity and inflammation. The deleterious health effects of chronic inflammation are very well known. On the non-physical plane, it manifests as withholding, lacking a capacity for intimacy, and characterological rigidity. Being undercharged means a person is not holding onto enough of his energy, allowing too much to move through too quickly to be effectively channeled into life-affirming pulsation and behavior. On the physical plane, this manifests as musculoskeletal flaccidity and listlessness. On the non-physical plane, it is manifest in underdeveloped personal boundaries and impulsiveness.

Perhaps because it's easier to see and measure, the energetics of the body have gotten much more attention than the energetics of the mind. But, the fact that there's no such thing as "mental acupuncture" doesn't mean that, in the quest for healing and greater health and wellness, we can neglect the energetics of the mind.

As the stresses of life challenge us and, in response, bodies manifest chronic patterns of musculoskeletal tension, minds, too, develop habitual ways of managing energy. Being "defensive" or "obsessive" or "explosive" all represent mental efforts to maintain an energetically unbalanced status quo.

When we "defend," we block the inflow of energy. When we "obsess," we store energy. When we "explode," we discharge energy in a mad rush.

While the ultimate healthy manifestation of the lifeforce moving through the human body is pulsation, its counterpart on the non-physical level is creative, purposeful, loving action. Creativity and being stuck are mutually exclusive. You cannot in the same moment be stuck and creative any more than you can, in the same moment, sneeze and have your eyes open.

Getting unstuck is a matter of channeling our lifeforce into greater creativity, purpose, and connection AND finding greater bioenergetic balance. Getting unstuck requires that we better balance the movement of energy through our bodies and engage in a greater degree of creative, purposeful, loving behavior. Getting unstuck means allowing the authentic being in each one of us to live freely in all its aspects and dimensions.

Just about anyone can benefit from getting unstuck. It's not something that's just for sick people. It's the rare person who isn't stuck, in some way, who doesn't suffer. It's even the rarer person who hasn't suffered enough.

The psychology I grew up with, the psychology of Freud and his intellectual sons and daughters, is fundamentally fatalistic.

Freud created psychoanalysis not as a way of helping restore capacity for greater joy and aliveness, but, rather, as a way of making the essential "unlivableness" of life more "livable." How inspiring is that?

Creative, life-affirming action is what we need to get unstuck, not resignation to the inevitability of our continued suffering!

In fact, when you're trying to get unstuck, it's best not to think of yourself as sick, either, because thinking of yourself as "sick" or "damaged" is helping to keep you stuck! Thinking of yourself as "sick" is like a negative affirmation. It's reminding you of your limitations, reiterating what you can't do and what's not possible.

If you are a therapist reading this, I'd also suggest that thinking of your clients as "sick" brings up a similar caution. While you might have to come up with a formal diagnosis to file an insurance claim, thinking of someone as, simply, "depressed" or "suffering from post-traumatic stress" doesn't tell you anything about how the person is managing his energy, so it's not going to tell you anything about how to help him (or her!) get unstuck. If you don't help him to get unstuck, you're just treating the symptoms, not the underlying cause. Help the person get unstuck and you really help him start to heal.

But why, we need to ask, would anyone get stuck in the first place? Getting stuck seems antithetical to life. Bad for the body, bad for the mind, and, frankly, bad for everyone around us, too.

Simply put, what causes us to get stuck is fear.

Fear of punishment. Fear of not being loved. Fear of failure. Fear of reprisal. Fear of abandonment. Fear of losing control. Fear of change. Fear of pain. Fear of pleasure. Fear of fear. Fear of life.

It is very interesting to look at what happens when a person is in fear. Breathing becomes more rapid and shallow. Muscles get tense. More stomach acid gets secreted. Hearts begin to beat more quickly. Thoughts become more rigid and obsessive. Adrenaline, norepinephrine, and cortisol, the three primary "stress hormones," get set into motion to help prepare us to "fight or take flight." The sympathetic nervous system gets activated to help us cope with the impending danger.

But what if, as is so often the case, the impending danger is more imagined than real? More a function of our imagination than our circumstances? I might worry about being punished for something I did (or didn't) do, but am I being punished at this very moment? I might worry about not being loved, but am I loved now? I might fear not being able to handle change in my life, but how am I handling things right now? Etc.

Truth be told: when it comes to fear, the mind is the conductor and the body is the train. The brain can't tell whether, or not, the pictures I create in my mind of certain gloom and doom are real. That's why scary movies scare us! And if those pictures we create are sufficiently negative, and sufficiently rehearsed, the nervous system goes into "chronic" mode and we develop static patterns of mental and musculoskeletal rigidity.

Some might call such patterns of static mental and musculoskeletal rigidity *sympatheticatonia*, i.e. a chronic activation of the sympathetic (fight or flight) nervous system.

I call it "being stuck."

Being stuck feels bad. Muscle tensions hurt. There's considerable evidence (in the work of Dr. John Sarno, for example) that most back pain—one of the commonest medical complaints in the world—is the result of "stress-related" muscle tension. And isn't "stress" just another word for unresolved fear? What about gastro-intestinal problems? When the sympathetic nervous system gets activated, more stomach acid gets secreted.

The fear that underlies being stuck might even help to make us fat. Because, when that same sympathetic nervous system is activated, metabolism slows and fats get stored rather than burned. There was even a study done years ago that suggested the reason why the French can eat their legendary high-fat diet with all kinds of cream and butter and baguettes and wine and maintain their relatively smaller waistlines is that they don't tend to eat in fear. While Americans look at a plate of rich, buttery food and immediately become anxious about calories and weight gain, the French look at that same dish and think, "Merveilleux ! Semble délicieux!"

Activity of the sympathetic nervous system is associated with inflammation, with disturbed glandular activity, with increased heart rate, and elevated blood pressure. Too much sympathetic activity weakens the immune system, puts stress on our internal organs, leads to pain, fatigue, and may contribute to obesity, as well.

Chronic fear is an equal-opportunity destroyer.

And what of its psychological effects? Anxiety, depression, insomnia, chronic anger, violence, marital problems, sexual dysfunction, drug abuse, eating disorders. The list goes on and on. Being stuck—a manifestation of chronic fear—gets expressed in a virtual smorgasbord of emotional, psychological, social, and existential problems.

Fear causes distress. But that is not at all to suggest that our "fear mechanisms" have no positive value. In a moment of real threat or danger, the mechanisms of fear alert us, heighten awareness, sharpen our vision, improve concentration, energize us. Any, and all, of those things may be critical to averting real danger, or just to surviving the horrible, scary things that can really happen in life.

But when the boogey man isn't lurking around the corner, when there is no real fire blazing, or terrible words being spoken, or guns being brandished, or threats getting made, or doom about to descend upon us, being stuck in fear just makes us miserable and leads to destructive behavior (which is sometimes directed towards others, as well as to ourselves). In fact, most of the destructive things that people do—abusing drugs, attacking others, over-eating, procrastinating, giving too much of ourselves, tolerating abuse, etc.—get triggered by fear and our efforts to ward it off.

Fear is what underlies being stuck and is at the root of all human suffering. To reduce our suffering, to get us on a more life-affirming path of healing, movement, learning, and pleasure, we've got to get unstuck. And getting unstuck often requires a willingness to confront our fear.

3

Making the Unconscious Conscious

ONE OF FREUD'S greatest contributions to human knowledge, and the thing which, perhaps, more than anything else, signified his genius, was his explication of the realms of the unconscious mind. His seminal work, "The Interpretation of Dreams," heralded the modern era of psychology, as it introduced to the world the idea that much of our behavior—and our problems— is rooted in a mysterious, virtually hidden, aspect of our mind—the unconscious. Freud went on to explain that the way to learn about the unconscious was to explore the world of our dreams. In our dreams, Freud believed, we'd be able to find the answers to our deepest questions and clarity about our motivations and desires. Doing so would help us to find greater peace in a world which was fundamentally fraught with conflict.

Over the many decades since Freud's passing, extraordinary advances have been made in psychology, neuroscience, psychophysiology, physics, and biology which have deepened our understanding of the universe and the nature of sickness and health. That said, Freud's belief in the importance of the unconscious to our understanding of human behavior has withstood the test of time. And one of the prevailing challenges for psychology and psychotherapy has been to find more efficient ways of making the unconscious conscious.

The basic problem to working with the unconscious is one of access. How does one explore that which is, by its very nature, hidden? And not merely hidden, but guarded by armed sentries, surrounded by a moat filled with snakes, and located at the far reaches of a badly drawn map filled with all kinds of twists and turns. It certainly sounds like a daunting task, doesn't it?

Moreover, we don't any longer have the luxury of time as in the days of Sigmund Freud and Carl Jung. When they were offering psychoanalysis to the denizens of Vienna and Zurich, all of life's activities took place at a relatively much more relaxed pace. Their patients came in to see them several times per week and often stayed in treatment for years. Expectations were quite different in a time prior to fast cars, cell phones, and instant karma.

Yet the fundamental task remains the same: help people understand the reasons for their suffering and offer them a set of tools for developing new ways of coping and thriving.

I'm humbly going to propose a new paradigm for accessing the unconscious and making it conscious. And that new paradigm rests in a single concept which offers up a fresh take on the mind/body relationship:

The body represents the unconscious. Whatever we need to know, whatever we need to understand about ourselves, to help us unravel the fears that keep us stuck, and which we might not otherwise be able to access, might be found by exploring our experience of the body.

I've already mentioned Wilhelm Reich as a major influence. While Freud was undoubtedly the great genius of the unconscious, Reich was, just as undoubtedly, the great genius of the mind/body relationship. He was, perhaps moreso than Freud, the grandfather of modern-day psychotherapy, for he was the first therapist to get his patients up off of the analytic couch and into a chair. Reich believed that it was only through being able to observe a person's posture and patterns of movement, eye contact, respiration, and his various twitches, vocal intonations, and manifest tensions that he could get an understanding of the patient's character.

For Reich, understanding character was key to understanding his patients and their underlying motivations and habitual patterns of responding to both their inner lives and the demands of the outer world. Did the patient hold himself well upright, with a firm grounding and sense of himself, or did he effect a slumped posture that suggested one of resignation and vulnerability? Did she make good eye contact? Was there significant tension around her eyes and mouth? Did his voice sound reedy, as if it were somewhat "choked off" at the throat, or was it more resonant? Did he appear to be breathing fully, or was his respiration shallow and restricted? Did she appear to be angry, or passive, taciturn or garrulous, fearful or trusting? Reich was the first psychologist to take note of such phenomena and make those observations central to his therapeutic work.

The body can reveal what would otherwise be hidden. So can dreams, of course. But dreams can, likewise, remain hidden. Some people can't remember their dreams well enough to allow for any useful analysis. And one can never be sure that, when reporting, or recording, dreams that they're not forgetting, or embellishing, the original content.

The body, on the other hand, doesn't lie. Absent bonafide underlying disease or deformation, all of the "symptoms" we develop in our bodies are psychophysical; they're all reflections, if not manifestations, of underlying psychological conflicts, defensive patterns, and efforts to cope with unmet needs, unfulfilled desires, and unresolved grief, pain, or fear.

But that doesn't mean the aches, pains, and chronic patterns of dysfunction in the body are not real. Suffering is suffering. The fact that your back pain may be the result of chronic emotional tension—rather than the result of a slipped disc or a fractured vertebra—doesn't mean that it is any less worthy of attention and care. I find efforts to dismiss so-called "psychosomatic" complaints as illegitimate simply because they can't be explained in terms of genuine physical trauma or disease disrespectful and counter-therapeutic. If we're going to utilize the body as a royal roadmap to the unconscious, we've got to begin with an attitude of respect. If a person knew of a better way to cope than to develop a pattern of musculoskeletal rigidity, he would have chosen it. Nobody wants to hurt. It's just that most of us didn't grow up with the tools to live a fully healthy, vital, empowered, conscious life and had no idea that, if they didn't have good, effective ways of dealing with their feelings, they might wind up paying a painful physical price.

If what we want to do is help ourselves, or help others to heal and learn and grow, we have to approach the problem with curiosity rather than with judgment. And we need to remember that the "mental" or "emotional" foundation of what would otherwise appear to be a "physical" problem is unconscious. No one makes a conscious decision to develop a stomach ache as a way of coping with stress.

We might also keep in mind that we don't develop dysfunctional patterns because we are stupid. We develop them because it's expedient, because it's what we're used to, because it's effective as a means of distracting us from underlying emotional challenges, because it's what we learned from our mothers and fathers, and because we don't know any better.

And it might also be worth considering that we develop chronic pain and patterns of suffering in our lives—unconsciously— in order to create opportunities for growth and learning.

This is, I think, a very important concept. We all have things to learn. We all have things to heal. We all have unconscious minds that could be more fully explored. Pain, distress, dysfunction, stuckness—these aren't just "problems." They're opportunities. Pain gets our attention. And if we pay sufficient attention, we're typically rewarded with a great opportunity for insight, growth, and healing.

An idea that I've always found compelling is that of the spiritual warrior. Holding the "spirit" as our attitude towards life and the beliefs by which we live—rather than as a word signifying any kind of religious idea or agenda—the spiritual warrior is a person who is constantly striving to become a better version of himself. Rather than going into battle with other people, he goes to into battle with who he has been. Rather than using swords and guns and fists, he uses awareness, insight, and courage. His goal is not to conquer, but, rather, to improve, not to vanquish an opposing soldier, but to overcome the limits of his own ego.

As a spiritual warrior, any problem I have is an opportunity for healing, growth, and learning. And as a therapist, any problem of yours that you bring to me is an opportunity for your healing, growth, and learning. Clinical assessment and diagnosis have their place, but the real joy for me—and, hopefully, the real joy for you—comes in supporting your growth as a spiritual warrior.

The spiritual warrior welcomes the chance to make what's been unconscious conscious. He (or she) wants to understand and, hopefully, better manage or overcome his fears. He wants not just to get over his symptoms, but also to get unstuck.

Judgment is one of the real enemies of the spiritual warrior. While pain can point one in the right direction, judgment can make the journey more arduous than it needs to be. Judgment blocks insight, and without insight, there is no growth and healing.

In curiosity, we ask of our pain, "What might I learn about myself from you?"

In judgment, we admonish ourselves for our stupidity, our indolence, our mistakes.

Years ago, I was judgmental about people in pain. Having been blessed with a strong immune system and a propensity to stay active, eat a healthy diet, and the great good fortune to live in a beautiful, pristine environment, I entered my 40s in excellent health. I took no medications, had never suffered a significant malady, recovered quickly from minor aches and pains, and was, as the old expression went, "fit as a fiddle."

When I'd meet a client my age, or a bit older, who suffered with the very common ailment of back pain, I'd say the right, compassionate things but, silently, to myself, carry on a very different sort of conversation. I'd think to myself, "Well, maybe if you were to get up off the couch, stop drinking so much beer, lose a few pounds, and hit the gym now and then, you'd be much better off..."

I was judgmental, rather than curious. I might have been able to offer up a few recommendations for managing stress or using self-hypnosis to control pain, but there was just no way

I was really going to be able to help that client heal. My judgment of him as "lazy" precluded my taking him on a deeper journey into his unconscious and the prospect of really helping him to get unstuck.

Fortunately for me, I got my comeuppance.

In my early forties, I undertook to install, by myself, a large air conditioner high up on the wall of our master bedroom. (In hindsight, I suppose that "needing help" was another thing I'd come to associate with laziness!) The task proved to be more than I'd bargained for.

As I climbed up the short ladder, heavy A/C unit in my arms, I twisted to hoist the behemoth up into the hole I'd cut into the wall. And wham! I was riveted by a powerful electric current that coursed down through my back and into my legs. My god did it hurt. While I was, somehow, able to get the AC unit into its compartment, I wobbled, fell, and wound up writhing on the floor in excruciating, burning pain.

It was some time before I could get up off the floor, walk around, and regain my equilibrium. Eventually, I went to see a doctor and got diagnosed with a herniated lumbar disc. And, for a good part of the next several years, I was one of those "guys in his 40s with back pain." Is it worth mentioning the irony here?

At first, I was judgmental. I berated myself for my "macho stupidity." I was angry. I was irritable. I was becoming someone I'd never wanted to be. And then, fortunately, I came to my senses. I remembered that I am a spiritual warrior, not a victim, that my pain was not an impediment to living my life, but potentially a key to greater self-understanding, and I began to heal.

Along with engaging in a rigorous course of physical therapy, chiropractic care, and acupuncture, I came to confront my worst fears about survival and took an honest inventory of my priorities. I explored what drove my refusal to ask for help when I needed it, which compelled me to look (yet again) into my troubled relationship with my father, my stubbornness, and the insecurity which drove my relentless need to be seen as "in control and on top of things." Eventually, the pain vanished and the MRI report showed that my damaged disc had healed.

And I discovered within myself a genuine compassion for people in pain.

Even when "real stuff" happens to our bodies, there is the potential to utilize our body experience to access the world of our unconscious. Rather than ask, "How could you do such a stupid thing?" we can ask, "What might this pain be trying to tell you about yourself and your healing?"

Again: curiosity, not judgment.

And let's not forget that body pain isn't the only language with which the unconscious communicates. What we often call "body language" has a rather large vocabulary. Posture, hand gestures, the resonance of our voice, the quality of our eye contact, breathing patterns—these are all part of the lexicon of the unconscious.

Have you ever wondered what posture suggests about underlying unconscious needs, feelings, and conflicts? Ida Rolf understood that posture—the alignment of the body in time and space—resulted from the effects of physical trauma and gravity.

Injuries occur in every life and, as the body heals, the connective tissues (fascia) tend to shorten and thicken. Gravity exerts a constant dynamic tension: we strive to hold our bodies upright while the force of gravity tends to pull us down. These two phenomena, according to Rolf, result in posture shifting and the body getting misaligned around its natural center of gravity. And I would be remis not to mention the role of inheritance, too. We are all genetically endowed with certain tendencies in the ways we look, move, and act.

But there is more to the picture. Posture represents not just an accumulation of injury, gravitational forces, and inherited traits. It represents the ways in which we hold ourselves in this world and the unconscious choices we make about how to cope with our fears, desires, and conflicts.

Think of what is usually considered to be the ideal male body. Shoulders back. Chest out. Waist small and taut. "V-shaped" upper body. Posture is "ramrod" straight.

While people might find that kind of image attractive, there's certainly no evidence that such a body is any healthier, less vulnerable to injury or disease, or less likely to break down than any other. It would follow, then, that the development of that kind of posture is not driven by a biological imperative.

The "ideal male body" hasn't evolved to help perpetuate the species. The desire to be thought of as sexually attractive certainly has something to do with it, but study after study has actually shown that characteristics other than a "V-shaped upper body" have far more to do with male romantic success.

What I'm going to suggest is that posture is also, or perhaps even mostly, a reflection of our unconscious efforts to manage our emotions and project an ego-syntonic image to the world (i.e. an image that reflects our self-beliefs).

When I was a little boy, Charles Atlas represented the "male ideal." He (not his real name, of course) developed a system of physical training and a network of fitness centers which promised to transform young men "from 97-pound weaklings to Greek gods." It was one of the most memorable and successful advertising campaigns in history.

I find the "Greek god" aspect particularly interesting. For what distinguishes a "god" more than anything else? Size? Strength?

No. It's "power." Gods are "in control."

Thus, the real, fundamental motivation for striving to achieve that muscular, V-shaped body with the ramrod-straight posture is the desire to feel in-control and to project an image of tough invulnerability. There's nothing wrong with, or necessarily pathological about trying to appear invulnerable, but only someone who has an unconscious insecurity and/or feeling of vulnerability would have that kind of concern. The attempt to conquer one's insecurity or feelings of vulnerability by adopting a hardened veneer isn't necessarily destructive, but it's got nothing to do with healing, with getting unstuck. Rather, it has something to do with silencing the unconscious, which speaks to us through the bodily experience of emotion—anxiety, pain, grief, anger, sadness, joy, excitement, etc.

The word "emotion" is an interesting one. When you look at the etymology of the word, you find references to "movement." Emotion represents energy in motion. Our feelings represent our experience of the lifeforce, the ch'i, the prana, moving through our body. The pleasantness or unpleasantness of the feeling is a matter of how we interpret the sensations. To the extent we are in touch with our emotions, life seems fully alive within us. To the extent we're out-of-touch, life is dull.

Key to emotional aliveness is breathing. Breathing is the primary way in which lifeforce enters the body and gets discharged. We experience this in-flow and outflow as feeling. Sometimes, feelings are pleasant; sometimes not. But, again, without feeling, without emotion, there's no sense of being alive.

We all try to limit unpleasant emotions. Anger, anxiety, sadness, pain are all unpleasant. Yet, they are (for good or ill), an important part of life. And, as we've already noted, they're vital to the language of the unconscious. Digging through and confronting such unpleasant emotions is often a necessary part of the process of getting unstuck.

The primary way we strive to keep unpleasant emotions under control is by not breathing fully. We limit our breath in an effort to limit our feelings.

Imagine you wake up in the middle of the night to get a drink of water. Stumbling through the dark on your way to the kitchen, you accidentally stub your toe. It hurts like hell. But, not wanting to disturb anyone else, you choke off your scream.

How do you do that? You stop breathing! You suck in a big breath, clench your teeth and your fist and you don't exhale. You know, instinctively, that if you were to let yourself exhale at that moment, your exhalation would be accompanied by a loud yelp of abject pain. You don't allow yourself to exhale until the initial mad rush of pain diminishes.

Here's another example: a young child begins to throw a tantrum. Her mother becomes frustrated. Yelling, at first, she pleads with her child to stop. The tantrum continues. Crying and screaming. Upon reaching the limit of her tolerance, the mother tries a different tactic. She tells her child, "If you stop crying and screaming right now, I'll give you some candy!" Upon hearing this, the child's attention gets piqued. She loves candy and makes the immediate decision to shift her behavior. And what does she do to stop crying and regain emotional control? She takes a short series of inhalations and doesn't exhale. Within a few moments, mom stops tearing her hair out and the child is happily scarfing up a bowlful of M&Ms (and no, I'm not recommending candy as a panacea for childhood behavior problems).

It would be easy to provide numerous other examples of situations in which we make efforts to keep our feelings under control. Being able to control our emotions is vital to us being able to function in an orderly society. But many of us learn that keeping emotions under control is more important than allowing ourselves to feel them and express them and that's not the truth at all. As the old expression goes, "there's a time and place for everything." Allowing one's self to fully experience and express a rush of sadness or anger might not be appropriate in a public forum, but might be necessary in a more private, intimate circumstance. Discernment requires not just the ability to limit our experience, but also a capacity for full expression. Difficulties on either side of the equation cause problems.

Now, back to that ideal male body with the tight abs and the puffed out chest....He might look great, and all, and he may be able to deadlift 1120 pounds, take a bullet in his arm without flinching, and wrestle a grizzly bear to the ground. But I'll tell you one thing he probably can't do: he probably can't complete a full breath.

I'm not suggesting that he can't breathe enough to give himself all the oxygen he needs. Of course, he can do that. But what he can't do is take the kind of deep breath that allows for a person, upon exhalation, to more fully relax. Because, to do so, his abdomen would have to be able to move freely and, well, the guy's got rock hard abs. "Rock hard" is the opposite of "moves freely."

The diaphragm is the main muscle of breathing. Sitting under the lungs, it separates the chest cavity from the abdominal cavity. Upon inhalation, the natural arc of the diaphragm is to swing downwards into the abdominal area. On the one hand, this requires that the abdomen expand; on the other hand, this movement allows for the lower aspect of the lungs to fill more completely with air. Upon exhalation, the diaphragm snaps up, as the abdomen flattens and air is pushed back up through the trachea and out.

Tight abdominal muscles—"washboard abs"—may look sexy, and all, but they don't allow for the complete downward swing of the diaphragm. Only the upper aspect of the lungs can fill completely. This certainly might allow a person to get the energy he needs, but it won't allow for a complete relaxation of the system. That's not a good thing. Being able to relax is important. Relaxation isn't merely restorative. It is essential to having the kind of full emotional experience which is often needed in the process of getting unstuck. To be able to feel fully, we've got to be able to breathe fully. And anything that gets in the way of breathing fully, of feeling fully, is only helping to keep us stuck.

If the experience of our body—essentially, our emotional life—represents the unconscious trying to communicate with us, then the efforts we make to limit, tightly control, or "cut off" from our feelings are antithetical to insight, growth, and healing. You can't get insight, growth, and healing without good communication.

Good communication, like all good things, begins with love.

In so many ways, "love" is another word for "truth." If I love you, I tell you truth. If I feel loved by you, I show you the truth of who I am. It's not necessarily easy to do, but it is a simple thing. Loving means (among other things) telling the truth. If I love you, I'll tell you the truth. And, if I love myself, I'll be honest with me.

In every relationship, there's an opportunity for learning. Something to learn about someone else, of course, but also an opportunity to learn about ourselves. You are my teacher and my student. If we teach each other with love, it can be, to borrow a phrase, like our own little course in miracles.

Acting in love—telling the truth—can be difficult. Scary. A lie or a deception might get exposed. Someone might get hurt or feel angry or disappointed. I might have to admit to needing help. Or to feeling insecure. You might have to admit to wanting to end a relationship. But if I don't tell the truth, I stay stuck and no one learns a thing.

Appreciating that there is value in every life experience is a loving act. Getting hurt, betrayed, deceived feels awful, but the momentary pain of such experiences can get eclipsed by the lessons that might be learned.

Years ago, I went through a painful period of self-doubt. My professional practice had slowed. The bills were starting to pile up. With some sense of relief, I was offered, and I accepted, a proposal from a local medical doctor to become part of his new, but already thriving, medical center. The offer came with significant financial incentives, which certainly was appealing, with two daughters at university and Hawaii's notorious "paradise tax" looming overhead.

"Larry" was younger than I, very bright and energetic, and his MBA, coupled with his MD, gave him serious cred as a potential healthcare business powerhouse. I'd felt excited to be hitching my financial wagon to a bullet train. I'd noticed Larry's arrogance, narcissism, and the condescending tone with which he treated his secretaries, aides, and associates, but I paid that little mind. He and I were "partners" in an exciting, lucrative, new venture, and he'd been treating me well. I ignored the stomach aches I'd begun to have nearly every day I spent at the Clinic.

I hadn't then realized that those stomach aches might've been a message from my unconscious. The ka-ching, ka-ching of my personal cash register, coupled with increasing amounts of wine every night with dinner helped to keep me blissfully narcotized to the sociopathy in my midst. Then, things took a sudden turn.

Larry had negotiated a very lucrative contract with a major local insurance carrier. My role was that of designing and supervising a treatment program while Larry's role was to manage the business and the medical needs of the patients. We assumed a shared responsibility for conducting the outcomes research which the contract had demanded. The net profits generated by the contract were to be split equitably upon its completion and I was to be paid handsomely thereafter as a permanent consultant to the program.

I worked diligently to help ensure our success, ignoring those stomach aches while striving to deliver a quality service to our patients and staff. As far as I knew, Larry had been doing the same.

But then, as the contract came to a close, and to my great dismay, and then anger, there was no money for me. Larry had, quietly and over several years, drained off tens of thousands of dollars as unsubstantiated "overhead" expenses. There was no evidence that these funds had gone anywhere other than into Larry's bank account. It might have all been legal, but it sure as hell felt like he'd embezzled a lot of money which would otherwise have gone to me as a share of the profits. Moreover, I found out through one of the patients that Larry had manipulated the research data. That just added professional embarrassment to personal injury and threw the integrity of the entire project into ethical despair. Eventually, there were lawyers. Nothing ever got resolved.

I was hurt, angry, bewildered as to how anyone, especially a licensed physician pledged to uphold a code of ethics, could conduct himself in such a way. Sure, I'd been aware of his peacock character, the coldness with which he sometimes treated others, and had heard some troubling stories here and there. But this? This was beyond anything I'd imagined. How could I have possibly known when I'd hitched my wagon to that bullet train, that it was heading for a crash?

I engaged in a lot of self-recrimination. How could I have been so stupid? Why hadn't I seen this coming? What kind of a schmuck was I not to vet this guy more thoroughly?

Perhaps the more important question to ask, the one I should have asked a long time before, was "What is this stomach ache trying to tell me?"

Maybe, if I hadn't gotten so caught up in the financial aspect of things and paid better attention to my unconscious as it was getting expressed through my body, I might've saved myself a lot of grief. I might've gotten unstuck more quickly from a sticky mess. Maybe the feelings of anxiety and disgust that lay under the stomach aches had been worth paying attention to all along.

I knew that those stomach aches weren't just about eating too many canned tomatoes or drinking too much espresso. But that's what I used to tell myself and others.

I'd always had a "sensitive stomach." I can remember on a few occasions coming home from elementary school with a stomach ache and my mother giving me a little bit of Crème de Cacao as a remedy. Looking back, it was probably the alcohol in this pleasant tasting liqueur that did the trick. The spoonful of liqueur calmed down my sympathetic nervous system and, for the moment, at least, quieted my unconscious voice.

When I say that I "knew" the truth about my stomach aches, what I mean to convey is that, in my "heart of hearts," I knew that canned tomatoes weren't causing all my problems. I didn't eat enough canned tomatoes, or drink espresso frequently enough, or do anything self-abusive enough to account for the grumbling and churning and "indigestion" that would often trouble me.

"Heart of hearts" is an interesting expression. As with "the gut," we draw upon an anatomical reference to express an experience of consciousness. Both expressions refer to the revelation of deep inner truth. "I know in my heart of hearts" or "I feel in my gut" both mean "you're about to hear what I really think and feel." These expressions have been around for hundreds of years, suggesting that the role of the body as a vehicle through which to access the unconscious has been understood intuitively, at least, for a long time (as have all the ways in which we delude, distract, and avoid).

Many people have asked me, "How do you know when you're dealing with or expressing your real truth and not just fooling yourself?" All I can say is this: The truth will set you free. BS will keep you stuck.

As for my situation with Larry, it would have been easy for me just to see myself as a "victim," as someone who got manipulated and stolen from by a clever criminal. But where would the insight, growth, and healing be in that? After all, a "victim" can only meet one of three fates: get victimized yet again, get rescued, or become a victimizer. None of that has any appeal. None of those outcomes brings with it the prospect of healing, of getting unstuck. We don't learn a thing from living in the so-called "victim triangle."

It took me a while to get it, but I finally got that the stomach aches were alerting me to danger, encouraging me to take better care of myself, and, most importantly, to trust that my path ought to be guided primarily by love, truth, and integrity rather than by my inherited fears of survival (as seems to be true for many children and, even, grandchildren of immigrants, the pursuit of wealth is a way of trying to secure membership in a society in which you don't otherwise feel accepted and secure. Ironically, many of us achieve financial success, but continue to worry about our security).

I still get the occasional stomach ache "for no apparent reason."

But now, I ask the right questions.

Back aches, stomach aches, headaches, muscle tension, insomnia, restless legs, stiff necks, all the ordinary aches and pains of life, may, of course, be indicative of real underlying dysfunction or disease. Each of us seems to have our favorite places to somaticize. But if it's not about bruises, fractures or illness, and if we're willing to explore them rather than ignore them, these "symptoms" can provide us keys to our unconscious and, ultimately, to getting unstuck. Unstuck from moribund relationships, unstuck from toxic people, unstuck from the shackles of our own fears, unstuck from our perceived limitations, unstuck from chronic self-defeating patterns.

Paying attention to these body-symptoms and asking what we might learn from them rather than just what we might do to get rid of them requires some time and trust and diligence and intention, but there will be rewards. Making the unconscious conscious is essential to getting unstuck.

4

The Tyranny of the Familiar

A **CLIENT OF** mine many years ago—I'll call her "Elizabeth"—came to see me for help with her anxiety. She'd had difficulty falling asleep, a persistent tension in her upper back, problems concentrating, and complained of a general feeling of impending doom. She'd recently been to her family physician and received a clean bill of health. But, she'd also received a prescription for Xanax, a commonly prescribed anti-anxiety medication, which she'd admitted to over-using.

Elizabeth was in her early 40s, pleasant, divorced, lived alone, and was financially comfortable as she had a successful career going as a real estate broker. She had friends, including a steady romantic partner, and no psychiatric history. But she had a striking physical characteristic: bright blue eyes which seemed almost frozen in a startled, wide open expression of fear. She had the proverbial look of a "deer caught in the headlights."

The second time she came to see me, as she dropped her large handbag onto the floor and plopped herself down into one of my big easy chairs, a paperback book accidentally spilled out of the bag. It was "Salem's Lot," by Stephen King.

I asked Elizabeth if she'd been enjoying the book. Her eyes widened even more than usual and she answered excitedly, "Oh, I love Stephen King. Don't you?"

What Elizabeth said she enjoyed so much about Stephen King's books—"Salem's Lot," especially—was that they are "so scary."

She went on at length about how much she loved scary books, scary movies, scary rides at amusement parks, and how she'd hoped that someday, soon, she'd be able to go sky-diving "because it seems really scary."

I found the dialogue fascinating. Here was a woman seeking help for what was, clinically-speaking, an anxiety disorder, a problem she'd claimed had troubled her for years, who, in fact, spent a lot of her free time scaring herself!! Did Elizabeth realize that, while she could, and needed to, do things to soothe her anxiety, to calm herself down, to relax, she was, instead, keeping herself hot-wired much of the time with frightening imagery (and caffeine)?

At first, Elizabeth found my query irritating. She became angry with me, and defensive. "Millions of people love scary books and movies," she argued, "and it's not like they're all needing therapy because of it."

"You're right," I agreed, "and there's nothing wrong with scary books. I've enjoyed a couple of Stephen King novels, myself. He's a terrific writer with an extraordinary imagination. But, if you're a person who struggles with anxiety, who can't sleep and needs potentially addictive medication to relax, it might be worth looking at how your regularly exposing yourself to anxiety-producing stimulation is contributing to your problems, rather than helping you, and what might be underlying that self-defeating choice."

Upon further exploration, we discovered that Elizabeth had struggled with anxiety her entire life. She couldn't remember a time when she'd felt completely at peace or completely safe. She had no idea why. Anxiety, it seemed, was, for Elizabeth, her default mode. It was, in a strange way, how she was most comfortable. Being anxious kept her "on alert" and ready to run at the first sight of danger. And, as she made very clear, the world was, for Elizabeth, a very scary place.

Elizabeth didn't report anything unusually disturbing about her childhood. She described her family as "intact," she had an older brother, there were no extraordinary dislocations, disruptions, or other trauma. She had "no idea' why she would have suffered with anxiety her whole life. "I come from a good background," she said repeatedly. "I had a good normal childhood."

But then, during our fourth meeting, something else emerged. Elizabeth reported that, just before leaving her home to come to our session, she'd had a phone conversation with her father. "How'd it go?," I asked. "Oh, OK, I guess…like usual. He'd been drinking so he kind of jumped all over the place…"

"Your father was drunk?"

"Oh, yeah, as usual. It's not as bad as it used to be. But he still drinks a lot. We've all just gotten used to it."

I asked if it was true throughout her childhood that her father was often drunk and, if so, what was that like for her.

"Well," she said, "it didn't really affect me that much. He'd usually come home drunk. He and my mom would fight a lot about his drinking but it's not like anything really bad would happen. Sometimes, there'd be a lot of screaming and I would just go up to my room and shut my door. I think he might've hit mom once or twice. But nobody ever got badly hurt. It's not like there were cops, or anything. A lot of my friends had it worse. It was a little scary, sometimes, but, no one has a perfect childhood, right?"

Right. But, almost as soon as she said that, Elizabeth's mood shifted. Her eyes looked down, then straight out at me with a pleading, puzzled look. "Maybe I did feel scared a lot when I was growing up."

"Yes," I replied, "and maybe you got so used to being afraid as a child that you've unconsciously sought out reasons to be afraid throughout your life because feeling afraid is so familiar."

At that moment, Elizabeth began to cry. "It's all I've ever really known," she sobbed. And her healing had begun.

It is one of the great ironies of life that we will tend to recreate in our adult lives the kind of environment we got used to in childhood. And, by environment, I mean emotional as well as social. Elizabeth had unconsciously over many years, recreated, and maintained within herself, the kind of uncertain, insecure, unsafe feeling she'd gotten used to growing up in a family environment marked by alcoholism, violence, and turmoil. She didn't do this because she's stupid. She did it because it's what was familiar—and what is familiar to us, even if it's uncomfortable, is what feels safe.

The late, great comedian, Buddy Hackett, described this phenomenon in a much lighter-hearted, but equally poignant, way.

Hackett liked to tell a story about his experience upon being drafted during World War II. Going through his basic training, he was no longer eating the rich, fatty food he'd gotten used to in his mother's kitchen growing up. One day, he showed up at the infirmary to get medical attention. "What's the problem, soldier?," the beleaguered doctor asked the young recruit.

"My stomach doesn't hurt," replied Private Hackett. "My whole life, I've had a stomach ache. Today, I feel fine. Something must be wrong."

In other words, when you're used to feeling bad, feeling good can feel bad.

We're all creatures of habit. We learn from a very early age to keep engaging in behaviors that get reinforced with praise or material compensation, bring us pleasure, or help us avoid discomfort. As we repeat these behaviors over time, the association between the behavior and the reward gets stronger.

At some point, we develop both brain circuitry and musculoskeletal patterns that anchor these behaviors in the mind/body as habits. The behaviors eventually become routine, effortless, unconscious. The greater the reward associated with a habit, the more firmly established the habit becomes. The habits we associate most closely with survival are the most powerful, and deeply entrenched, of all.

For Elizabeth, maintaining a near-constant state of fearfulness was critical to her survival. Keeping her sympathetic nervous system turned on helped to keep her alert to impending danger and ready to take flight upon feeling threatened. And what she'd learned early on in life, when her mind and body were most receptive to new learning and developing new patterns, is that the world is a scary place. Her father's alcoholism and violence were a constant threat to the peace and tranquility of the family home. While his drunkenness was predictable, the violence was not. "Will dad be in a bad mood when he comes home today?" "Will he and mom get into another nasty fight?" "Will things be OK?"

Those were all questions little Elizabeth couldn't answer, and not knowing made her feel insecure and scared. In time, that fear became a habit, became her way of approaching life, coping with stress, surviving. Her anxiety might have made it difficult for her to sleep and concentrate, but it was a familiar feeling that she'd come to associate with survival, and that gave her some sense of control. Reading scary books and watching horror movies weren't just entertainment for Elizabeth, they represented ways of her recreating a childhood marked by volatility and insecurity and reminding herself over and over again of the need to be alert and stay in control.

Corinne was in her early twenties, single, and "depressed." She'd been referred to me by another therapist who'd "given up" trying to help her. Corinne was bulimic and had been binge-purging virtually every day since high school. From a wealthy local family, Corinne had been well-educated in an elite private school and carried herself with poise and an air of sophistication. But she couldn't seem to avoid getting into relationships with abusive men. Her last boyfriend had broken her wrist.

"He was so good looking," Corinne recounted, "but he liked things a little rough in the bedroom....bondage stuff. I didn't really like that, but what's a girl to do? Most of the time, it was ok. I figure a little pain just goes with the territory. But one night, it got a little out of control.... If he hadn't broken my wrist we'd probably still be together. But I have my limits." She laughed seductively. " I draw the line at broken bones."

I pointed out the incongruity of her laughter. "Well, crying is a most unattractive quality, isn't it?," Corinne averred. "And if a girl isn't attractive, what has she got left?"

I noted Corinne's numerous references to "attractiveness" and the importance she seemed to place on physical appearance. I asked if it were important to her that I find her attractive.

"Well, do you?," she replied.

"Let's not make this about my feelings, Corinne. Let's make this about you," I responded. "Is it more important to you that I find you attractive or that I understand you?"

"No one's ever asked me that before," she answered. "Understand me? Yes, sure, of course. I'd rather be understood. But I don't know if I've ever felt understood."

"What's that been like for you, Corinne, to go through your life without ever feeling understood?," I asked.

"It sucks. It really sucks." Corinne was on the edge of tears.

"Can you say that again, Corinne, even louder? Take a big breath in and let the words out as you exhale."

"It sucks," Corinne yelled, "It really fucking sucks. I hate it."

Corinne went on over the next few sessions to reveal that she'd come from a family in which "appearance was everything" and "making a scene was a big no-no." Her father, whom she loved but also "feared," was a prominent member of the community who'd repeatedly emphasized the importance of the family image. Corinne was expected to perform well at school, have the "right" group of friends, and, especially, look and act like the perfect daughter.

She realized that her bulimia had begun at age 15 after her father told her that "if (she didn't) lose a few pounds, no man is ever going to want (me)." She'd felt "devastated" by his comment, but never let on, never spoke about it to anyone.

She just "went on a diet" and, after she'd heard about another girl at school who was bulimic, she began vomiting every night after dinner. Eventually, the vomiting "took on a life of its own" and became her way of relieving stress, calming herself down, and, especially, of coping with angry feelings. She'd also become quite sexually promiscuous, sometimes with boys who, she acknowledged, "were not very nice."

"I'm really a very angry girl," Corinne acknowledged," I've just learned to keep it hidden. I mean, in my family, we never fought, never got out of control. I don't know if anyone is really happy but, like they say, "it's better to look good than to feel good."

And being with men who cared more about how she looked than about how she felt, more about what she could do to make them happy than about what they could do to make her feel happy, was just part of the role she'd been raised to play. "Oh God," she said during one of our sessions, "I've become just like my mother!"

Habits can be useful, necessary, and positive. But they can also get in our way. They can contribute more to our staying stuck than to our vitality, growth, and healing. Maintaining a posture of fearfulness might help us to avoid danger, but it can also make it impossible for us to trust. Without trust, intimacy becomes impossible. We might be safe, but we're also alone. Pretending that "everything's alright" might have been important to help keep the peace in our families growing up, but sets us up to be hurt, exploited, and disrespected by others later in life.

The survival habits we develop in childhood are truly mind/body phenomena, as they are manifest in both the ways in which we think and the ways in which we hold ourselves and move. These habits form our character armor. The primary purpose of armor is to protect us, but, as with any kind of armor, what protects us might also tend to keep us constrained— immunized not just to the dangers we might imagine and perceive, but also to change and growth. Armor that is too rigid keeps us stuck.

The idea of character armor was first conceived by Wilhelm Reich. While many of his other bioenergetic concepts have always been controversial, his book, "Character Analysis" has had a profound and lasting impact on psychoanalysis and psychotherapy. In that book, Reich explored the mind/body connection in a radically new way, as he articulated the various patterns of "armoring" and how they impacted therapy and the work of helping people to change. Fundamental to the practice of character analysis was the making of unconscious patterns of psychological rigidity and musculoskeletal tension more conscious. By bringing "stuckness" into a patient's awareness, Reich encouraged his patients to explore their deepest pains and fears and, ultimately, allowed them to make healthier more life-affirmative choices.

Elizabeth wasn't stupid. She was unconscious. She had no idea that marinating, as she did, in scary stories and images was helping to recreate the same existential circumstances with which she'd struggled as a child. Corinne wasn't dumb. She wasn't "a masochist." But she was unaware that denying her true needs and feelings was both leading her into degrading sexual relationships and causing the bulimia that was endangering her life.

We do, as the old expression goes, have to be careful about what we wish for because we just might get it. And we have to be especially careful about what we imagine and what we project out into the world. Because the world out there just nods.

Whatever I really think I am, whatever I really think I'm worthy of, the world of other people, that great field of infinite possibility, says "Yup." The abusive husband, the failed career, the misery, and, likewise, the wonderful marriage, the great success, the happiness, are reflections of the self-image we maintain and project out into the world. Respect attracts respect. Fearfulness attracts fearfulness. Love attracts love.

The so-called "law of attraction" tells us that we receive from the universe what we imagine and affirm. We attract the perfect new lover into our lives by visualizing and affirming that she's on her way. We make attracting that new lover less likely by imagining rejection and thinking of ourselves as unworthy or unattractive. Financial success begins with positive vision and belief. Healing rests on a foundation of faith. The "law of attraction" is certainly not infallible. It does not bring to light all the mysteries of the universe. But I think its basic veracity is unquestionable. I've seen few instances over the course of my life of a distrustful person finding real happiness in a relationship or a person who didn't really believe in himself finding success in his business. And I've certainly known a

number of people whose efforts to overcome personal hard-
ship would never have been successful had they not cultivated
a positive attitude to go along with their hard work.

The one twist that I would add to a discussion of the Law
of Attraction is that I think we don't just have to be careful
about what we wish for, or, as Kurt Vonnegut once said, "what
we pretend to be." We've also got to be careful about what
we prepare for. If my expectation is that the world is a dangerous place, I will prepare to be attacked. I'll adopt either a
resigned or combative stance towards the world around me
and will be disproportionately concerned with staying safe.
This resigned or combative stance—characterized, in part, by
a disempowered, passive posture in the former and a pugna-
cious, prideful bearing in the latter—will, in turn, attract a
world that suits our expectations. Victims attract victimizers
and vice versa. Because she continued to carry around with
her the negative beliefs and musculoskeletal tensions she'd
developed to cope with a childhood that demanded she be
"pleasant" and accommodating at all times and help maintain the image of "a perfect family," Corinne really couldn't
help but attract partners who cared little about her needs
and feelings. She also had few resources for resolving conflict, since she'd grown up in a home where conflict was,
simply, swept under the rug. Her bulimia represented a cock-
eyed, and ultimately self-destructive, way of expressing all
the anger and frustration she'd learned to keep hidden. The
disrespectful, sometimes violent, lovers reflected Corinne's
sad sense of her own self-worth.

If you want to break free of old patterns, you've got to—literally—break free of old patterns! The habits we developed in childhood to deal with our emotions, cope with neglect or abuse, maintain a sense of control, survive whatever we had to endure, and maintain some biopsychosocial equilibrium are encoded in the psychological circuitry of our minds and in the energetic circuitry of our bodies. It is within this circuitry we find echoes of what we learned from childhood about ourselves, what to expect of other people, how to get what we want, how to connect and protect, and how to cope with pleasure, pain, anger, fear, joy, and sadness.

Getting unstuck is a mind/body experience because both mind and body are involved in, and were involved in, getting stuck in the first place. When a child learns not to cry, it's a mind/body experience. He develops negative thoughts and images associated with crying and habitual patterns of muscular tension to hold back his tears. The mind and the body are two aspects of a single being, one reflected in the other, connected with the other, and always interdependent.

We might certainly develop mind/body patterns in childhood that are positive, life-affirming, and don't need any review, repair, or rehabilitation. Maybe they need celebration! I hope we can all identify some positive patterns in ourselves. But suffering is an indication that we've been holding onto a mind/body pattern that is getting in our way and has, at the very least, outlived its usefulness. The dangers we might have actually been subject to as a child might only be virtual dangers now that exist only in our imaginations.

It makes no sense for us, as adults, to remain as if we were still children struggling to cope with family circumstances beyond our control. Maybe crying would lead to our getting scolded again, or worse. But is that still a legitimate fear? Might something which we once needed to get us through now threatening to bring us down? I'm reminded of that old expression about the cure being worse than the disease.

As I've already mentioned, healing does require faith. I'm not pointing to faith in any religious or supernatural sense, but rather to faith as a belief in a process. Change can be challenging, even scary. We never can be certain of what's on the other side of the wall. We're not caterpillars who can shed our skins. We've got to work with what we've got, which means we've sometimes got to stretch—and stretching can be painful.

But when you learn to stretch just so much at a time, breathe into it, and find that place of greater ease that's really always available, you'll find that there's much more pleasure than pain to be had. And that getting unstuck is more than just possible. It's also a wonderful, thrilling, liberating experience.

5

Love & Fear

EACH ONE OF us goes through challenges in life. We face real dangers. We get hurt. We hurt others. We have disappointments. We fail. We lose. We make mistakes. What distinguishes the good, or successful, or happy life from the life of suffering and misery isn't a simple matter of "luck" or "fate." It's a matter of choice. The Buddha isn't smiling because he's gotten everything he's wanted. He smiles because he's gotten what he's gotten. Life is what it is. As the great spiritual teacher, Ram Dass, taught us, all the stuff that happens in life is "grist for the mill." It's all there to serve us. What we do with what we get is the most important thing. We might not get to choose whether, or not, we get sick, or lose a loved one, or get rich or get old, but we most certainly do get to choose whether, or not, we allow those experiences to strengthen and deepen and enrich our experience of being alive. Victims only see what the pains and frustrations of life do to them. Masters of life ask what those same pains and frustrations might do for them.

The kind of mastery I'm describing is available to anyone willing to do the work of getting unstuck. That work begins with becoming a spiritual warrior. As I'd described earlier, being a spiritual warrior doesn't require any kind of religious identification or practice. There are spiritual warriors who are deeply religious and others who are atheist. Some who meditate and some who do yoga. Some who are vegan. Some who'd eat a vegan (just a joke). There are spiritual warriors who'd never in a million years think of themselves as spiritual warriors. To me, anyone willing to honestly confront his fears in order to find greater peace and be a better version of himself is a spiritual warrior.

We all have fears. We might not all have nightmares, but we all have our fears. It's not just those of us who had a horrible childhood or other traumatic experiences. We all have "insecurities" and negative expectations. We've probably all had moments, at least, when getting overwhelmed with our fear made life seem like a living hell.

What a great expression that really is. A "living hell." It suggests there's a "living heaven," too, doesn't it?

If the proverbial "living hell" is a life of intense anxiety, a "living heaven" would be one of great love.

A life of great love would be one of great giving and receiving, but neither one more than the other. Just as there would be no inhalation without exhalation, there'd be no receiving without giving (and vice versa). Love is the yin and the yang and the yang and the yin. Love creates the possibility for new experiences and learning. Fear, on the other hand, creates limits.

It is in the very nature of fear to create more limited experience. Our focus narrows, we get ready for action. All of our energy goes into fighting or taking flight. We look to survive, not to thrive, and to rely on the safe and the familiar even if it may not be all that safe. Fear makes it more difficult to learn, and less likely we'll try something new, because when we're in fear, we become more defensive, more focused on doing than on receiving, more impulsive.

Fear, in mind and in body, makes us more inflexible. And that inflexibility will be expressed bioenergetically and psychologically, in body and in mind.

If you look at fear from the perspective of the body, it's an acute activation of the sympathetic nervous system with associated biochemical changes that affect the respiratory system, the circulatory system, the musculoskeletal system, and the way we respond energetically to the world around us. In a moment of fear, we ready ourselves to take flight or fight by getting our systems "overcharged." Muscles contract to sustain the increased tension and provide that greater burst of speed or strength we might need at the time. But chronic activation of the fear cycle leads to chronic muscle tensions that reduce our overall bioenergetic flexibility, i.e. keep us stuck.

Psychologically, in a moment of fear, we become more acutely focused. As our field of awareness narrows, so does our consideration of detail and nuance. Our world instantaneously becomes simpler: black or white, right or wrong, good or bad. In a moment of real danger, we need that kind of simplicity and clarity. We need to channel all of our resources into the task of survival. But when the fear response becomes chronic—because we keep scaring ourselves—we get "stuck" in survival mode. That makes us defensive, less available, more resistant to new experience and learning.

Chronic fear gets anchored into the mind/body as character armor. The armor begins with those little things we do that help to keep us safe in the moment but, with repetition, evolve into something that keeps us stuck in old patterns of thought and behavior. And being stuck in old patterns of thought and behavior isn't just uncomfortable—it's the basis of our suffering.

Life is about movement. Pulsation. Emotion. Change. Learning. Growth. These are what life is all about. These are what distinguish the feeling of being alive. Without them, life is stale and dull.

When we breathe in, we take in energy. This charges our system, gives us energetic fuel. When we exhale, we discharge excess energy and the system relaxes, ready to begin the next cycle. This is illustrated in a simple diagram:

Charge → Activation → Discharge → Relaxation

Chronic tension in our respiratory system leaves us bioenergetically out of balance. If the system can't discharge fully and relax, it tends to stay overcharged. If it can't charge fully, the system will stay undercharged. Either way, pulsation gets flattened; life gets diminished. Feeling fully alive requires giving and receiving, taking in and letting out, venturing forth and standing still. Some chronic bioenergetic tension may be necessary to allow for us to maintain a sense of order and control in our bodies, but too much just helps to keep us stuck and limits our experience of life.

Likewise, chronic fear leaves us psychologically out of balance, as well. It is one thing to do what we need to do to stay safe and protected; it is something else entirely to remain hidden behind a curtain of fear.

Boundaries help to keep us safe and establish a sense of our own identity. What's within the imaginary circle I draw around myself is "me" and everything else is "not me." When boundaries get created out of love, they're firm and flexible, neither too rigid nor too porous. I have a good sense of who I am and where I stand but I'm open to new experience and ideas. When boundaries are created out of fear, they're either too rigid or too easily crossed. Fearful people either tend to wall themselves off from the world around them or lose themselves in the experiences of others. Their sense of self is more fragile, less grounded. They're more stuck in what's familiar to them, and more concerned with their survival rather than with their aliveness.

Basically, what we are in fear of is emotion and new awareness. In our bodies, fear manifests as chronic bioenergetic tension that keeps us from being able to feel. In our minds, fear manifests as chronic defensiveness that limits our capacity for new experience. Fear keeps us stuck in old patterns.

We experience the movement of energy through our bodies as feeling, as emotion. The chronic muscular tensions we develop serve the purpose of binding energy, of holding, or containing, feeling which would otherwise move through us and get felt. This principle would apply to any kind of emotion—pleasurable or painful—which we won't, or can't, let ourselves feel. And we all have emotions that we don't want to feel.

The range of possible human emotions is broad: anger, sadness, fear, pleasure, excitement, disgust, love, surprise. They all involve different sensations, evoke different images, memories, and associations. To each emotion, we've attached a meaning, a valence, a degree of receptivity. To the emotions we've come to associate with negative consequences, we've developed armoring. The armor helps to keep us from feeling and/or expressing the emotions freely.

Fear and love are the most basic, perhaps the most fundamental, emotions. The associations we make with them are probably the most deeply ingrained and consequential. This doesn't mean that anger, pain, pleasure, and surprise don't matter. But it does suggest that a more fundamental relationship with love and fear exists. Some might argue that love and fear are the "primary" emotions, the roots of all feeling. They certainly are at the roots of all armoring.

We develop armor in fear. Fear of being punished, ridiculed, shamed, ostracized. Armor functions as blocks to awareness and self-expression. We armor ourselves against emotions we can't let ourselves express and thoughts we can't accept. While love welcomes the full expression of our being and acceptance of life, fear helps to contain and give us a sense of control over the parts of ourselves we can't accept and the dangers we expect from the world around us. Love represents expansion of our sense of self and holds within it the promise of transcending our current state of being. Fear is all about maintaining and protecting the status quo.

Ironically, armor interferes with our joy and laughter just as much as with our sadness and tears. If you can't cry fully, you can't laugh fully, either. The same armor that protects us from feeling pain also limits the extent to which we can experience pleasure.

Which brings us to the matter of sexuality.

Of all the controversial ideas Wilhelm Reich got criticized for, none was more controversial than his beliefs about orgasm. To Reich, the capacity to orgasm was the *sine qua non* of bioenergetic health. Orgastic potency, as Reich called it, was the most important measure of a person's aliveness because orgastic potency was determined by a person's capacity for energetic charge and discharge. The orgasm, as Reich understood it, served the vital life function of discharging all of one's accumulated excess energetic charge. Without complete discharge via regular orgasm, the bioenergetic system remained in a chronic state of imbalance, either overcharged with too much tension or undercharged and relatively listless. Reich's "orgonomic functionalism" explains that chronic armoring is what causes the lack of orgastic potency. The natural flow of energetic discharge in orgasm gets short-circuited. The pleasurable experience of orgasm gets constrained in the sinews of the muscular armoring and distorted by a mind troubled by guilt and shame about sex. According to Reich, the lack of orgastic potency is crippling to a person's sense of aliveness and his capacity for love, work and the accumulation of new experience. Distortions of the natural energetic processes were viewed as contributory in problems of violence, compulsion, even cancer.

One can only imagine the degree of scorn such an idea received within the conservative intellectual circles of Vienna in the 1920s. Years prior to that, Freud had, likewise, been vilified for suggesting that the sexual lives of children was a worthy topic of psychiatric inquiry. Even after he emigrated to the United States in the 1940s, Reich, with his "radical" idea about the function of the orgasm, was slandered with contrived stories about "sex boxes" and masturbating his patients.

Unfortunately, one doesn't need to look very far to see that, even today, 75 years later, the idea that sexual pleasure is important to health and wellness continues to evoke ridicule, outright dismissal, scorn from the prudish and sniggers from the immature.

To discuss fully the value of sexuality and sexual pleasure, and all of the associated conflicts and controversy, would require a dedicated book, or three. Suffice to say that, in my experience, both personally and over the course of my 35+ years as a psychotherapist, I've come to believe that Reich was correct, at least insofar as a healthy attitude towards sex and a capacity for deep, loving sexual embrace are vital components of a healthy life. I would also add, however, and in contrast to Reich, that the concept of "orgastic potency" seems too narrow if what we're talking about is getting unstuck. I think that excess energetic charge can get released through crying, shouting, creativity, aerobic exercise, too, so getting unstuck doesn't require a focus on sexual release, per se. In my opinion, any kind of genuine energetic expression can work. The important factor might not be orgasm, but it may well be the capacity to surrender fully to our emotional experience, whether that is an experience of sexual pleasure or sadness, joy, anger, etc. Armor gets in the way of that and keeps us stuck. Armor represents a fear of being fully ourselves and a fixed way of responding to life.

Love, on the other hand, helps to get us unstuck.

Love isn't easy. Much of the time, it's the more challenging choice. We have all learned not to love ourselves completely, not to value all of who we are. Even the most loving parents can impart to their children a somewhat mixed message in this regard. "Big boys don't cry" and "children should be seen and not heard" aren't mean-spirited messages but they can, nonetheless, have a big impact on a child's capacity to become a fully at-ease adult. We all learn, even in loving families, that some things about who we are are not acceptable. We might be "too sensitive" or "too fat" or "too loud" or we might "ask too many questions." Whatever those negative, unloving messages might be, we tend to believe them, or, at least, act like we believe them, and they have an impact on how we wind up dealing with our feelings, desires, and preferences.

Authenticity becomes at least a bit of a struggle for every one of us, as we grapple with traits, qualities, emotions, and interests that we learned, growing up, were unacceptable, or worse. Our efforts to armor ourselves against them serve as tensions within us that keep us in conflict with our true nature.

As spiritual warriors, we must go into battle with those tensions and seek breakthrough into our true nature. But the spiritual warrior's primary weapon is not a sword or a rifle. It is love.

"Can I love my anger?" "Can I love my passionate, hearty laugh?" "Can I love my sensitivity?" "Can I love my body?" "Can I love myself enough to say 'No'?" "Can I love myself enough to say 'Yes'?" "Can I love myself even though I've made a mistake?" And what would "loving myself" be like? It is easier to say "I love you" than to act in a loving way.

Love gets defined in a myriad ways. Each of us has our unique ways of defining it, talking about it, expressing it. One of the words that I use to define love is "truth." Loving means telling the truth. We may not be inclined to tell the truth in all situations and to all the people in our lives. There may be times when not telling the truth is the best choice. But those situations are relatively rare. Speaking generally, I think we have an obligation to tell the truth to all the people we love, starting with ourselves.

Telling the truth can be difficult. Like I've said, love is not necessarily the easier path. We might encounter truth that disappoints, or hurts, or turns our world upside down. But, if you're looking to heal something, or solve a problem, you've got to start by telling the truth. You've got to start with love.

You can no more build a house on a shaky foundation than you can heal a troubled soul with bullshit.

Acting with love is also the most powerful way of attracting love from the world around us (just as, I would add, being fearful is the most powerful way of attracting fearfulness). That's what the law of attraction teaches us. Treating ourselves and others with love—rather than with fear—is the best way of bringing more love into our lives.

Too often, love gets mistaken for "giving." A willingness to give of one's self to another is certainly a part of loving behavior. But love means "receiving," too. Yin and yang. Yang and yin. In the matter of treating other people with love, I'm not just referring to being kind, or being generous, or being of service. Those are all loving acts, for sure. But it's only one side of the proverbial coin. As I'd suggested earlier, we enter into a relationship as both potential teacher and student. It is in the very nature of any relationship for us to give and be given to.

Some people certainly seem to just get given more than others. But is that really the case? Might the Beatles have been right when they sang, "The love you take is equal to the love you make?"

I have a very dear friend who has had a very full life filled with great joys, adventures, amazing people, and material wealth. I used to wonder what he'd done to attract such great good fortune. Years ago, I learned the secret.

It was Rick's birthday. He and his wife invited a small group of us over to their home to celebrate. After dinner, we lounged in the living room, listening to music, joking around, doing what eight good friends usually do together at a party. Before it got too late, his wife, Annie, announced that it was "time for presents."

Upon hearing that, Rick politely turned down the stereo, picked up and moved their coffee table to the side of the room, then gracefully sat down in the middle of the room in a full lotus yoga posture. He smiled and said, "OK now...I'm happy to receive."

One by one, we each gave him a little gift. A t-shirt, a CD, a sweet. Upon receiving the first of his gifts, a CD, Rick smiled, and with a twinkle in his eye, said "thank you." Then, he got up and fed the CD into his stereo. Upon receiving the next gift, a colorful T-shirt, he immediately exclaimed, "Oh, boy," and put it on—right over the shirt he'd been wearing. Upon receiving the candy, he exclaimed, "Oh, boy," again, popped a piece into his mouth, then insisted everyone share in the treat. And so on, until he was wearing four t-shirts all at once and we'd all listened to a folk song, an electric blues, a few minutes of exotica, and finished off the candy. We all laughed heartily and had a great time.

And then it struck me. "The world has given so much to Rick because, at least in part, he receives so wholeheartedly. He makes everybody feel so good about giving to him. He loves generously, but also welcomes generously the love that people want to give him." An "aha moment" if ever there was one.

For most of us, this kind of loving attitude doesn't come easily. We struggle with trust, with acceptance, with our sense of worthiness. The wounds of childhood, and the rejections, losses, and failures we've endured through our life's journey have all left their scars. But obsessing about those scars, identifying with them, contributes to being stuck rather than to our healing and eventual freedom. Each of those scars has value. It has something to teach us about how to love ourselves or about how to love others. Finding out what those lessons are can take time and work. But that process also demands our love. Fear only conjures up judgment and prejudice. Fear can't help us gain insight or find greater acceptance. Only love can bring forth curiosity and an openness to deeper truths. And if love doesn't come so easily, we have to cultivate it. Read about it, ask questions, seek guidance, hang out with loving people, practice.

Consider that every single one of us gets wounded. Every single one of us wounds others. Hurting and getting hurt is as much a part of the history of mankind as the development of language. Our wounds, our scars, do not make us unworthy of being loved or finding peace. To the contrary, they may be jumping off points into a life of greater self-knowledge and understanding. Avoiding our wounds or pretending that they're not there just gives them more power. After all, it takes energy to avoid and pretend. That's energy that might otherwise be available for living.

Getting unstuck is about freeing up that energy, loosening the grip that those scars have on us, so that we might breathe more freely, feel more fully, and thrive rather than just survive.

Fortunately, we each have within us an instinct to move through fear and into love. It's our unconscious. The unconscious exists not just as a repository of emotional memory and unspoken desire, but also, and most importantly, as a source of truth. When the unconscious "speaks" to us through our bodies, or through our dreams, it's giving us an opportunity to make deeper contact with who we really are. Those tensions we feel in our bodies, those especially vivid or disturbing dreams we sometimes have, are meant to show us the deeper truths about our lives, those feelings, conflicts, and desires that we otherwise, out of fear, would avoid, dismiss, and neglect. The unconscious is really there to serve us, enlighten us, help us shift from fear to love, from stasis to movement, suffering to peace. Choosing not to pay attention to the unconscious helps only to keep us stuck—and ensures that we accumulate lot of "unfinished business."

"Unfinished business" is a term from Gestalt therapy which has become commonly used as a reference to anything we've left incomplete, unsaid, undigested, or unresolved. It actually goes against our nature to accumulate unfinished business. The archive of unfinished business we drag around with us is a constant source of anxiety that contributes to staying stuck.

Gestalt therapy derives its theory in part from Reich and in part from Gestalt psychology, which began with the study of visual perception. In simple terms, Gestalt therapy emphasizes the need to organize experience into a meaningful, completed whole, which, as the widely used expression suggests, "is often greater than the sum of its parts." Emerging experiences, which references anything that captures our attention, are either seen to completion or remain fragmented in our consciousness, sucking up psychic space and energy. Think about words that never get said, tasks that never get finished, feelings that never get expressed, interests and desires that never get explored. Such "incomplete Gestalten" are a constant source of anxiety and can become an unconscious obsession.

Years ago, when my father was a kid growing up in Brooklyn, he and his friends would go to the movies on Saturday afternoons. For a nickel, they'd get thrilled by the exploits of their favorite movie heroes like Buffalo Bill and The Lone Ranger. These serialized dramas were often called "cliffhangers," because each episode would, typically, end with the hero facing some great danger, like riding his horse over a fast-approaching cliff or trying to save the damsel-in-distress who's about to fall out of an open window. Just before the hero would meet his fate, the episode would end, leaving the kids with bated breath and sweaty palms—and with a fierce determination to be back in the theatre the following week. They just had to find out what happened!

Despite our natural urge for completion, and the distress that incompletion causes, we often leave things incomplete and undone. We don't make that phone call, pay that bill, write that paper, fold those towels, see that doctor, paint that cabinet, have that meeting. We don't pursue that dream. We don't cry those tears or let out that scream. We don't face the truth about that terrible loss or horrible trauma. Some unfinished business is more damaging to our lives and well-being than others, but all of it is destructive. Unfinished business gets in the way of new experience as it binds up our mental and physical energy. Not doing what we need to do can be exhausting.

Unfinished business serves to keep us stuck by being a constant source of anxiety. When we don't complete the things we need to complete—-especially those most important things that pertain to our welfare, our health, our most valued relationships—-we feel anxious. We feel "ill at ease." We don't sleep soundly. We overeat. And overuse. And overspend. We develop addictions.

Anxiety is like the psychological equivalent of muscle tension. Just as muscle tension can be a source of disabling physical pain, anxiety can be mentally disabling, rendering us unable to focus, make decisions, or relax. Chronic anxiety is also, like chronic muscle tension, less a sign of a "real" problem than it is a sign of our unconscious trying to get us to pay attention to the unfinished business in our lives.

Completing unfinished business needs to be a focus of anyone who is committed to getting unstuck. Breaking free of the cycle of fear that underlies being stuck requires that we stop doing things that keep ourselves in fear. Just as Elizabeth needed to stop reading the scary books that kept her on-edge, anyone who struggles with being stuck needs to commit to living a life of greater love and less fear. Treating one's self with love often means taking practical steps to do what you know you've got to do, what that inner voice of your unconscious is exhorting you to do: talk to a therapist about your grief or shame, call your dad, clean out your closet, come out of the closet, quit your job, do your job, see a doctor, start that project, pay your taxes. In other words, complete your unfinished business.

Choosing love over fear means honoring yourself and your healing by telling the truth of your experience and doing what you really need to do, no matter how challenging or upsetting that might be to your status quo. Positive thinking and affirmations and prayer and meditation and journaling and t'ai chi and eating more vegetables are all good things to do. But, whatever you do, the most important thing you can do is to choose love, not fear. Only love is empowering. Only love will get you unstuck.

6

Boundaries

IF YOU WERE to look up "personal boundaries" in Wikipedia or Psychology Today, you would find references to the rules, limits, and preferences we exert in establishing our own sense of identity. The common understanding of the personal boundary is that it's like an invisible line we draw around ourselves to help distinguish me from you. The boundary is the place where "I" ends and the rest of the world begins, the point of contact between ourselves and our social environment. The boundary has both physical and psychological importance, is multi-dimensional, and touches upon many aspects of life.

Most of the time, our personal boundary operates in the background of our consciousness. Like the anti-virus software on your computer that silently scours for problems and doesn't make itself known until a threat shows up, the personal boundary doesn't tend to make itself known until it's needed. In the presence of great love, divinity, or beauty, the sense of "oneness" we feel is as if the personal boundary has melted away. The capacity to let go of our personal boundary momentarily, or, at least, to keep it in the background, is vital to profound spiritual experience, to heightened creativity, and to sexual intimacy.

At other times, the personal boundary needs to be more active. Imagine arriving a few minutes early at a movie theatre. There's just a small handful of people seated and many empty seats around. It is our sense of personal boundary (and our awareness of the boundaries of others) that compels us to sit away from, rather than next to, a stranger. Or maybe, at a social gathering, a sense of our boundaries drives the choices we make about whom we talk to, whose hand we shake, whose cheek we kiss—or whom we let kiss us.

Each of us has some sense of what physically "close" feels like and, consequently, of what "not close enough" and "too close" feel like, as well. This is also an important boundary function. When our physical boundary isn't respected, we are discomfited. More extreme boundary violations can leave us traumatized. A sense of good, healthy boundaries helps us to feel safe and in-charge of our lives and our personal space. But what makes for good healthy boundaries?

When that line we draw around ourselves is too thick and rigid, we're safe, but our capacity for intimacy and for new experience gets limited. If I'm threatened or just don't want whatever life might be presenting me, a thick, rigid boundary makes it easy for me to say "No" and keep myself safe. But, if what's being offered to me is love, is tenderness, my thick, rigid boundary will get in the way. On the other hand, if I've drawn my boundary line too faintly, I may be wholly receptive to the love that's being offered me, but unable to ward off danger.

A healthy boundary is neither too dense, nor too porous, and is flexible, not rigid. A healthy boundary is a filter, or a membrane, which allows for absorption of what is good and welcome, but functions as a barrier to what is perceived as toxic, or unwanted. This would apply especially to feelings, preferences, and demands of other people, as we need to be able to allow in that which brings us joy and enhances our experience of life and keep out that which causes undue stress or injury.

But the personal boundary functions as more than just an interface between ourselves and the world around us. It also helps to define who we are by helping us to contain and give some shape to our energetic character. A healthy boundary helps us not just to filter out what is incoming from the environment but also what might flow outwards from us towards the environment. Without a sufficiently firm boundary, it is more difficult to focus and sustain concentration, keep one's own impulses in check, and express one's feelings appropriately. An insufficiently firm boundary may also lead to chronic lethargy or indolence, as energy is always leaking out through what is, essentially, a poorly developed container.

But the overarching problem faced by the "underbounded" person is one of disempowerment, typically marked by a fundamental attitude of "passive resignation" toward the world and a pervasive feeling of being a victim. In other words, the "underbounded" person tends to see himself, and conduct himself, as if other people are in charge of his life and there's nothing he can do about it.

Raymond was 41 years old. He and Karen had been married for 14 years and had two children. Raymond had been referred to me by his chiropractor, who had been seeing him for a persistent lower back pain of unknown etiology which had been unresponsive to treatment. Raymond had no psychiatric history, reported that he "only sometimes felt a little depressed," and said he was happy with his successful law practice and his marriage and family life. He didn't have friends or much of a social life, but felt alright about that because he had "such a wonderful wife." He was bright and articulate but also kind of flat, as he spoke in a rather monotonous tone that portrayed little emotion. I was struck by his physical appearance, as he was quite tall, much wider at the hips than at the shoulders, with a soft, protruding belly, and by his demeanor, which was passive, withdrawn, and diffident. He also had a habit of apologizing frequently, as if he felt sorry for his own existence. He was "mystified" by his ongoing back pain, which had been bothering him for a few years, on and off, especially so because he'd recently bought himself an expensive desk chair that was "supposed to be good for lower back problems."

As Raymond had never spoken with a therapist before, and was skeptical of its value, he was reticent. Over our first few visits, he was relentlessly polite to the point of obsequiousness. He apologized again and again for not being able to remember parts of his personal history as well as his reluctance to discuss in detail the parts that he could remember. But he was more than happy to complain about his back, how badly it hurt, all the doctors he'd seen, the medications he'd tried, the sleepless nights he'd endured. He believed his back pain "must be a genetic thing" because his fathered suffered similarly.

After several visits, I was able to persuade Raymond to try a simple relaxation exercise. To my surprise, he responded very quickly and he seemed to enjoy the feeling. When he was in that more relaxed state, I asked him to close his eyes and pay close attention to the feeling in his lower back, to tune in and tell me as much about what he felt and what came into his mind as he possibly could.

Raymond described the tension and pain in his back as "like my bones and muscles are fighting with each other." But his mind, he said, was "blank." I pressed him a little further. "Can you, Raymond, remember the very first time you had pain in your back like that, pain that felt like your bones and muscles were fighting with each other?" At that, I noticed his lips began to quiver.

"What's happening in your body right now, Raymond?," I asked. "Can you let yourself exhale more fully?" As he did, the quivering became more intense. His eyes became teary and he began to whimper. I asked if it was OK with him if I just touched his chest with my hand and pressed slightly. To my surprise, he said it was OK. And, as I did, Raymond began to cry. After a few moments of tears and sniffles, he opened his eyes. "I remember the first time my back hurt," Raymond nearly shouted, "It was that first time that Karen got into trouble." By this point, he was sobbing.

After he regained his composure (and apologized for using up a bunch of tissues), Raymond told me about that "first time Karen got into trouble."

It winds up that Karen was severely alcoholic and had had to be "rescued" many times from bars late at night after she'd gotten herself into some "awkward" situations with other patrons. Raymond recounted in teary detail the first time he'd gotten one of those late-night phone calls and how "embarrassed and ashamed" he'd felt. With some prodding, he was able to acknowledge that he'd also felt angry at Karen. The back pain, he offered, "happened the first time that night but it's gotten even worse as she's continued to drink. She doesn't go out to bars, anymore. Now, she gets drunk at home and just gives me a hard time."

By the end of that session, Raymond said he felt some relief. He still had a long way to go in terms of his healing, his getting unstuck from his old patterns, building a firmer boundary, and making decisions about his marriage. But he'd never acknowledged the truth about this part of his life before—his deep anger and resentment towards Karen for her drinking—and he saw, for the first time in years, "some light at the end of the tunnel."

Raymond had been stuck in a common, debilitating pattern of mistaking for love his desire to protect Karen from his true feelings (and her own misery). Yes, he most definitely loved and cared for his wife. But his repeated efforts to maintain the status quo by sheltering her from his troubled emotions and pretending everything was OK weren't being made out of love.

Nor had Raymond been treating himself in a loving way, either. He'd been choosing to live a life of real pain and misery rather than risk really being himself—a guy who was, among other things, full of anger and resentment who wanted his wife to stop drinking, get her shit together, and be a good partner. Raymond had, like so many of us, been resisting the truth of his own life by adopting a posture of passive resignation toward it. It's as if he'd been, over the course of many years, saying to the world, "Do to me what you will. I give up." This posture of passive resignation represents how Raymond kept himself stuck in a long- term pattern of disempowerment and dis-connectedness.

Disempowerment happens when we disavow our anger and, in so doing, lose our ability to say "NO" to the things we don't want and render our personal boundary limp and ineffective. Anger can be destructive, but it is an essential ingredient to the formation and maintenance of the boundaries which both protect us and help us to contain and channel our energy.

Raymond's relative lack of energy—disempowerment— made it difficult for him to take necessary action to express his true feelings or effectively make demands on his wife because that kind of personal affirmation and assertiveness requires energy.

Disconnectedness happens when we get so wrapped up in the needs and feelings of others that we lose the sense of being connected to ourselves. Disconnectedness makes it impossible to form and maintain a healthy, vibrant relationship because being disconnected from ourselves makes it impossible for us to be authentic. If I don't know what I really feel and can't say what I really want, any relationship I form is going to be a proverbial house of cards. The slightest stress is going to cause it to come crashing down.

On the other side of the coin, the "overbounded" person tends to have trouble not just with letting in, but also with letting out, especially more tender feelings and needs, as emotions and impulses that really need to get expressed get held back, leaving the person in a chronic state of tension, both physical and psychological. While the underbounded individual may struggle with his vulnerability and lack of self-esteem, the person with boundaries that are too rigid is hard to reach and his sense of self is, if anything, overblown.

Unlike the passive resignation we see in those whose boundaries are too flimsy, the person whose personal boundary tends to be too stiff and rigid—-the "overbounded" individual—-communicates a very different message. Instead of saying "Do with me what you will," it's as if the overbounded person says to the outside world "No, I won't and you can't make me." His is not a posture of passive resignation but, rather, one of active defiance.

Terry came to see me after his cardiologist insisted he needed to reduce his level of stress. Terry was 47, divorced, and an accomplished jazz musician. He'd recently suffered a minor heart attack and had begun taking medications to thin his blood and lower his blood pressure. He was tall and thin, but quite muscular, and he walked into my office the first time with a kind of swagger, almost as if he were preening for a camera. He was very carefully groomed, without a hair out of place, and clearly took great pride in his appearance. He had an angular face, with steely eyes and a prominent jaw. "So, you're the great Dr. Orenstein," he said as he extended his out-stretched hand, "What, exactly, are you gonna do for me?"

When I explained to Terry that I'd have to get to know him a little better before I could even begin to answer that ques..., he abruptly remarked, "Get to know me better? What? Are you gay?" He didn't appear to be joking.

"No, Terry," I responded, "I'm not gay. I just need to know some things about you before deciding how I might be able to help. I assume you're not gay, either. Do you have a woman in your life?

"You mean a 'bitch?' No. No one in particular. You know they all just want 'more, more, more.' I'd rather fuck a whore than ever be married again. But (laughing to himself now), they're all whores. Aren't they?"

I remarked to Terry that he looked, and sounded, angry.

"Oh, I see what you're doing, DocTor OrenSTINE," Terry snarled mockingly, "you're trying to 'get me into my feelings', huh? Well, to be honest, yeah. I'm fucking angry. You'd be an-gry too if you'd ever been through what I've been through."

Terry then went on to tell a long story about his ex-wife having an affair with a fellow musician and stealing his money. Of course, he spun his yarn with a great deal of invective and a paucity of humility or insight. I'd imagined that he'd felt terribly hurt by his wife's behavior, but Terry never came close to acknowledging that.

At one point, I asked Terry if he understood what had gone wrong in his marriage and what role he might've played in its demise. He glared at me, raised his voice, sarcastically questioned whether I was implying that "this all happened because my mommy spanked me too much," then went on to curse out his wife a little more. After a few more minutes of grunting and spewing, Terry again called out my name in a mocking tone, snarled that I'd "probably lied" about being gay, then got up and left my office.

Needless to mention, I never saw him again.

The overbounded person, with his posture of active defiance, is tough to reach and he doesn't reach out. Personal problems are always someone else's fault. His being stuck in a defensive posture against the world, pushing out angrily so much of the time, may help to keep him safe (cuckolding ex-wives aside). But that safety comes at a steep price—isolation. Intimacy can be nearly impossible with the overbounded person, and connectedness to a larger community a great challenge.

Ironically, while the underbounded person and the overbounded person might seem to be complete opposites of one another—the former vulnerable and clinging to connection, the latter relatively impenetrable and remote—-they actually have quite a bit in common.

To begin, they are both stuck in a pattern of behavior which is inflexible and dysfunctional. The underboundedness of the passively resigned is no less a "fixed" way of responding to the world than the overboundedness of the actively defiant. Both patterns render a person impaired in his capacity to form and maintain healthy loving relationships. While Terry's overt anger saw him constantly pushing against the world, keeping people and more tender feelings at a distance, Raymond's inauthenticity, his incapacity to express his real feelings and needs, made him nearly as poor a candidate for a loving interdependent partnership as Terry.

Another way in which the underbounded and overbounded are more similar than different is that they both have a chronic problem with personal power. The underbounded person tends towards disempowerment. His lack of firm boundaries allows for too much of his energy to leak out, leaving him undercharged and lacking the energetic capacity to take needed action to fix what's broken in his life.

But the overbounded person—-and Terry provides a great example of this—-tends to try to disempower others, particularly by adopting a haughty attitude, acting with hostility, trying to intimidate, or by engaging in outright abuse. Two sides of the same coin, so to speak.

Both the underbounded person and the overbounded person also share a tendency to resist contact with significant aspects of themselves. The former tends to reject, deny, and distance himself from his anger. The latter tends to reject, deny, and distance himself from more tender feelings, like hurt and sadness. Both individuals are insecure; the overbounded just does a better job of covering it up.

Perhaps more than anything else, our boundaries, how we form them and maintain them in both mind and body, reflect our energetic character. We may, as individual human beings, be distinguishable by all kinds of physical and mental characteristics. But, the energetic imprint we make on the world is as important as any, and that energetic imprint is all about our capacity for giving and receiving love.

Underboundedness and overboundedness result from fear. Both patterns help to keep us stuck in fear and struggling with love. Both patterns result in suffering. Both are a reflection of a lack of trust in one's self and the outside world. Getting unstuck, recreating boundaries as more flexible, adaptable structures, requires confronting one's fear and finding one's love.

The integrity of our boundaries—their strength, firmness, and consistency—is a reflection of the degree to which they are maintained by love or by fear. Boundaries maintained in love are used to contain and channel our energy for positive purposes: to protect us in the event of genuine threat, to allow for us to feel and express emotion, to allow for us to connect with ourselves and the outer world, and to disconnect when that suits us. Boundaries maintained in fear protect us from imaginary threat, limit the degree to which we can feel and express emotion, and create barriers to contact with ourselves and the outer world. Boundaries limit pulsation.

Truth be told, few people are strictly underbounded or overbounded. We are all complex, multidimensional beings. Speaking in absolutes about virtually anything related to human life is too simplistic. It would probably be more realistic to think in terms of a trend: one or the other of under-boundedness or overboundedness tends to be predominant. It's also worth reiterating that boundaries are a necessity. Without a capacity to put some limitations on our experiences, both within ourselves and socially, civilization would probably wind up a swirling incoherent mess. But such an eventuality is, at the same time, unthinkable, because boundary formation begins at a very young age and is as natural an aspect of our development as is the ability to communicate.

Boundaries are not the problem. Boundaries not made and maintained in love are the problem. This brings us to the role of trauma and shame.

Trauma is a terrible event that caused a person significant pain, loss, or subjected them to the threat of death. It is not necessary for a person to have been seriously physically injured for an experience to have been traumatic. In fact, some say that trauma actually occurs in the moment just prior to the horrifying event, when the brain, in an act of self-preservation, initiates a "shock" response and shuts down all but the most essential life functions. When there is physical injury, especially when that injury results in long-term impairment, the impact may be intensified, and more difficult to overcome. But the psychological impact of trauma, which is what we are concerned with here, does not require a precipitating physical event to have a profound effect on a person's life. Most people "recover" or "rebound" from trauma well enough that it doesn't render them seriously impaired. But others suffer from extended bouts with "post traumatic stress disorder," which is a very real and, sometimes, crippling condition.

Even when trauma doesn't rise to a "diagnosable" level, it can have a profound influence on the development of personal boundaries. It's another thing that binds together the experience of the underbounded and the overbounded: trauma often has had an impact on both of them.

The underbounded individual fears letting go of a relationship. His fear of losing love and not getting it back may be so profound that no price for holding on seems too great to pay. This is, in fact, why an underbounded person will, so often, remain in an abusive relationship no matter the physical, emotional, or financial toll. The fear of being alone outweighs whatever the perils of remaining together. It's not just a question of confidence, or financial independence, or opportunity that keeps the underbounded person hanging on. In fact, many beautiful, desirable, wealthy people are stuck in abusive relationships. The culprit is the unfinished business of attachment trauma.

Attachment trauma refers to a special kind of loss early on in life, usually prior to age 2 or 3, when the young child is completely helpless and dependent on his caregiver, typically his mother. Physical or emotional abuse might be involved, but the essential ingredient in attachment trauma is that the young child has the experience of losing love and being neglected or abandoned. Mother withdraws her love, or disappears, or, by virtue of her detachment, avoidance, addiction, or dysfunction, leaves the young child with a deep insecurity that manifests in a profound need to cling to whomever, or whatever, might promise to fill the void. Unresolved attachment trauma will compel an individual to cling tightly to anyone who might offer him the love, comfort, security, bonding, and companionship they desperately crave, even if they have to tolerate a bunch of bad behavior along the way. And they'll resist feeling too angry, or doing anything to empower themselves, because conscious anger and greater empowerment would pose a threat to the relationship.

The underbounded structure develops as a result of unresolved attachment trauma and the efforts that the traumatized individual makes to get, and keep, the love that they fear will be taken away. This sets them up for a bout of anxiety at the mere thought of separation or even just temporary loss. Denying their own needs and feelings, "people-pleasing," and tolerating what would otherwise be intolerable is, for the underbounded person, merely the price of admission to a life spent not alone. The posture of passive resignation I've described is easy to understand when you consider the nature of the underlying trauma.

Overboundedness, on the other hand, results not from a fear of being alone, but from a fear of not being left alone. The underlying trauma was not marked by a loss of love, but rather, a loss of sovereignty. The overbounded individual was, as a child, subject to what I call enmeshment trauma. He wasn't abandoned; he was engulfed. Whether he was raised in an enmeshed family, which couldn't tolerate emotional distance or disagreement, or he was subject to extreme demands for intimacy (emotional or sexual) by a custodial parent, the child who grows up to be overbounded wasn't allowed his individuality, his own space, his own life. Pushing back against intrusion—with anger—became his one way of maintaining his sense of identity. It became his only way of resisting enmeshment. Allowing himself to surrender, to really share love, to be close with another person, became risky. So he developed the kind of armoring which would shield him from that. Offers of intimacy, of deep personal contact, trigger fears of engulfment, so he only enters into relationships in which he can feel in control. He attacks and intimidates not out of inherent meanness, but out of a fear of being annihilated. He's every bit as fearful as his underbounded counterpart. He just develops a posture that makes him seem like he's more secure and grounded than he really is.

The boundaries we develop, whether the ultimate pattern is in the direction of overboundedness or underboundedness, reflect the nature of the underlying fear. And the degree to which these boundary patterns get stuck is a function of the depth of the underlying trauma and the anxiety that continues to get evoked. Repeated losses will only help to anchor the insecure, clingy, desperation of the underbounded person and repeated violations of personal space will only serve to harden the aggressive defenses of the overbounded.

In both circumstances, shame also can play a significant role. It has been said that shame is a feeling of self-loathing. As distinguished from guilt, which refers to feeling distressed about what we've done, shame refers to feeling distressed about who we are. While fear is what causes us to develop boundary issues that complicate and impair our interpersonal relationships, shame gets in the way of our relationship with ourselves.

Shame results in losses that are intrapersonal: we resist contact with aspects of ourselves that bring us distress or that we associate with being "bad," "wrong," "dirty," or worse. This may refer to emotions, sexuality, preferences, interests, virtually any personal trait that might be subject to judgment. Shame can have a powerful impact on anyone and affords equal opportunity to the underbounded and the overbounded. Shame causes internal breaches in our sense of self, as if we construct boundaries within ourselves to separate out the "acceptable" from the "unacceptable." We are diminished by the feelings we won't allow and the needs and desires we won't let ourselves express. Our healing and growth are made more difficult by our resistance to embracing all of who we are.

Years ago, in a Gestalt therapy workshop, Anthony, a fellow trainee, was confronted by the workshop leader for "giving up being Italian." This was said in a good-natured way and referenced the common stereotype of the lively, colorful, animated communication style associated with Italian culture. The remark had followed the leader's failed efforts to convince Anthony—who was of 100% Italian heritage—to use his hands when he spoke and express himself in something other than a dreary, uninspired monotone. Upon hearing this, Anthony suddenly burst into tears and recounted the abuse he'd suffered at the hands of his Sicilian grandfather. It proved to be a painful, but liberating, encounter as it helped Anthony reconnect with a disowned part of himself to find some greater vitality and sense of self-worth.

Shame may be attached to any experience of failure, loss of dignity, or dishonor, but it is especially common in cases of trauma. Very often, a traumatized individual, whatever the nature of the trauma, itself, is left feeling not only torn up about what the trauma did to him, but ashamed of how he responded to it.

Truth be told, most people don't handle trauma well. Trauma is a sudden, unforeseen event for which no person would be prepared. No one goes into any situation with an action plan in the event of trauma. No world leader has ever given a speech in which he's said, "In the event that I am traumatized..." Trauma is, by its very nature, unpredictable. So no one really has any cause to be judgmental, or even critical, of the way in which someone may have responded to watching his buddy's head get blown off on the battlefield, or crashing his car into a telephone pole at 70 miles per hour, or getting molested by Uncle Ernie. And yet, the person who has been traumatized in one horrific moment in time may spend years suffering recriminative, abusive self-loathing for "letting it happen," "not seeing it coming," "not being able to fight back," and the like. This kind of shame can be deeply injurious and always makes the work of healing and getting unstuck more difficult.

A big reason why shame gets so often associated with trauma is that a common response to trauma is to freeze. People don't, typically, take evasive action in traumatic situations or take steps to escape it once it begins. To the contrary, they do nothing other than endure the trauma. That's because a moment of trauma gets mediated within the mind/body in a way that's somewhat different from how we react to pain or danger.

When faced with a threatening situation, our sympathetic nervous system gets activated and we wind up fighting or taking flight. When trauma blindsides us—-and we never do see trauma coming—-the parasympathetic nervous system gets activated in such a way that it causes us to freeze. Both our physiological and cognitive systems get de-activated. It's as if we suddenly stop breathing, stop feeling, and stop thinking.

The traumatized person doesn't fight back or run away because he's weak, or bad, or stupid. According to "polyvagal theory," at a moment of trauma, the dorsal aspect of the vagus nerve, part of our basic survival system, initiates an autonomic response of the parasympathetic nervous system that shuts the rest of the person's systems down. The heart slows way down, the breathing slows way down, the musculature goes flaccid, the mind dissociates. A person can't control this "freezing" in a moment of trauma. It's what he does to survive it. Chronic musculoskeletal tensions and dysfunctional boundaries are a common consequence. Much of the time, chronic shame becomes part of the equation, as well.

In my experience, recapturing the flexibility in one's boundaries requires not just the release of pent-up emotion, the resolution of fear, and a more loving and realistic re-framing of one's existential world. It also requires a willingness to encounter and accept aspects of one's self that have become "disowned" by decree of shame. Of course, sex and anger and stubbornness and any number of other human traits may have "minuses as well as pluses." But banishing to the netherworld of unconsciousness one of your given traits to avoid ever having to encounter its negative aspect deprives you of the opportunity to make use of its positive aspect. And that's self-defeating.

People who have unresolved trauma and shame need to have a trusted relationship in which they can tell their story. They need to learn that "freezing" was a normal, adaptive response to intense stress and not something to be ashamed of. They need to learn that anxiety is a part of every person's life and something that can be managed. And they need, like anyone else looking to get unstuck from old patterns, to ask themselves whether, or not, the defenses, strategies, habits, and ideas they developed long ago to survive still make sense today.

7

A Matter of Balance

A POSITIVE PSYCHOLOGY needs to be focused on personal growth and not merely on symptom removal. Psychological traits, even those which might be considered problematic, need to be understood as part of the whole mind/body gestalt. Each aspect of who we are and how we think and behave serves a function. It can be challenging to figure out what function that may be, but a positive approach always seeks the value in experience and always looks to enhance, not diminish.

Shouting might be considered rude and coarse, but if you can't shout at a child to get out of the way of a moving car, you might fail to prevent an avoidable tragedy. Every human trait has its place. The trait isn't the problem. Being stuck is the problem. Shouting at that child for not putting the box of corn flakes back up on the shelf may, indeed, be destructive. But shouting at him to step back up on the curb might help to save his life.

If we focus simply on getting rid of "unwanted" behaviors, we may wind up satisfying a diagnostic imperative, but we don't support a person's growth. The cure, as the old adage suggests, should never be worse than the disease. If we're not encouraging a person's growth—-if we don't take steps to support our own growth—-we're not supporting life. Getting unstuck is what supports growth. Free up a person from the prison of his old, habitual ways of dealing with his feelings and other people and, like a tree transplanted from a small ceramic pot to a field of rich soil, he'll flourish. It's the way of life.

Because psychological health and wellness can't be understood as merely an absence of illness, we can't apply a conventional system of measurement to gauge it. An absence or presence of some certain characteristic might be indicative of a problem and it might not be. Context matters in psychology. Make a sarcastic joke in New York City and people will laugh. Tell that same sarcastic joke in Honolulu and people will cringe. An arrhythmic heartbeat or an abnormal EKG points to illness no matter where you live, as would paranoid delusions or intractable depression. But psychological health doesn't just mean that a person doesn't believe he's the reincarnation of Superman; it suggests that he's fully engaged in his life, i.e. finding pleasure, value, and meaning in who he is and what he does, thriving, adapting, learning. Psychologically healthy people might sometimes get depressed or have a sleepless night or binge eat or argue with their spouse. They just spend most of their lives being at peace and value the distressed moments as opportunities to learn and continue their healing.

The keys to psychological health and ongoing personal growth are empowerment, adaptability, competence, and openness to new experience, not an absence of diagnosable mental illness. Shit happens in everyone's life and the only thing perfect about life is its absence of perfection. We all have flaws and things to learn. How we cope with what comes our way, the degree to which we can embrace reality with love or push it away out of fear is, in the end, what matters most.

Empowerment is the most fundamental energetic process. We take in lifeforce, get activated, discharge, relax, and then the cycle repeats. It is the core pulsation of human life. To the extent this cycle gets limited, we are disempowered. When we are disempowered, we lack the energy we need to deal effectively with life, and so begins a typically chronic pattern of limitation, if not withdrawal.

Disempowerment can happen as a consequence of an interruption at any point in the cycle. A person can get disempowered by not letting himself inhale thoroughly enough or by not engaging fully enough with the life that's being offered him (which are remarkably similar things, when you think about it). Or, maybe a person lacks the capacity to tolerate energetic activation (read: emotion), so his energy "leaks out," and isn't channeled into purposive, life-affirming activity. Or, maybe, he contains his energy so tightly that he just gets overcharged to the point of explosion. Each of these situations would require something different to bring the system back into balance.

Adaptability requires flexibility, the capacity to respond appropriately and effectively. To the extent a person is stuck in old patterns of coping with stress, their capacity to adjust to changing circumstances is impaired. I might have discovered, as a child growing up, that getting angry at my intrusive mother was the only effective means I had to keep some needed distance. Perhaps she tended to ask for too much every time we spoke about personal things. But maybe I tend to get triggered in the same way by my wife, and I get angry at her, even though her demands are not nearly so intrusive. Greater flexibility would allow for me to choose among a broader variety of responses and, thus, build my capacity for intimacy and become a better, more loving, partner.

Competence refers to one's confidence in being self-supporting, not in the financial sense (though that can be a factor), but in the sense of being able to treat one's self with love and respect. Asserting one's boundaries effectively, asserting one's needs, expressing feelings, affirming one's sovereignty, these are all part of being competent. You might also think of competency as being a reflection of one's self-esteem. It is hardly radical to suggest that self-esteem is a key to psychological health. Some might even say that it's the master key, that without self-esteem, nothing else you do to further your personal growth is going to matter. A negative sense of one's competency commonly manifests as a "victim mentality," which is so very limiting. Greater competence results from facing life's challenges, particularly social challenges, setting goals, and working to achieve them. Self-esteem comes from within. Everybody likes to hear nice, complimentary things. But what we tell ourselves is the most important message we hear. If that message is negative, we stay stuck and suffer.

Being open to new experience is, obviously, key to growth and wellness because it's key to acquiring new learning. Openness to new experience demands humility. This can be hard for some people, especially for those of us who have learned to cope by acting like we already know everything. Truth be told, no matter how smart, insightful, well-read, therapy-wise, or successful we might judge ourselves to be, there's always something new that's possible to learn about ourselves or the world around us, always something we've never really experienced before. Closing off one's self to new experience might be safe and might've been necessary at some earlier point in our lives. But staying stuck in that place means, well, it means you're always going to be in that place. And that's not what life is supposed to be about.

Coping well requires not that we never get triggered or never make stupid mistakes, or that we never fail. But it does require that we humbly realize it is all "grist for the mill." Life is, really, such a "mixed up, muddled up" crazy, unpredictable rollercoaster ride that believing "it's all here to serve us" is essential. Without that, a sense of humor is impossible and I, for one, don't even want to try to imagine a life without laughter.

It is easier to blame than take responsibility, easier to think about "unfairness" and "bad luck" and "your fault" than it is to be on the path of a spiritual warrior. It is definitely more challenging to ask of a loss or problem, "what am I meant to be learning from this?" or "how can this contribute to my healing?" than it is to play the victim. But blaming, bitterness, and not learning from one's mistakes is never the better alternative. Put another way, when that notable British philosopher, Michael Charles Jagger, wrote "you can't always get what you want, but you get what you need," was he, or was he not, tapping into a vein of universal truth?

You turn the keys to psychological health and open the door to psychological wellness with curiosity. Curiosity allows for us to see and understand things in new ways. Curiosity pushes us to ask about "why" something happens rather than whether or not it has any value. Curiosity presupposes that everything has value. A curious mind thinks of things as part of a great continuum rather than in black/white, either/or terms. Anger has a place along the continuum of human emotion. It is neither "bad" nor "good." Its existence proves its value. Yin and yang. Yang and yin.

Without contraction, there'd be no expansion. Without light, there'd be no dark. Without heat there'd be no cold. The judgmental mind emphasizes distinctions. The curious mind looks for commonalities. When we look for commonalities, we find that there is a time, place, and purpose for everything, and, rather than avoid and seek escape from life, we embrace its "full catastrophe." We seek to include, rather than exclude. A positive psychology realizes that not only does every virus have within it the seeds of its own destruction, but that within every system in conflict there can be found a place of balance.

In human beings, that place of balance, or, more accurately, of greater balance, is the centerpoint, and the goal of a positive psychology is to help people find that place. The centerpoint is the place along the bioenergetic continuum which allows for the greatest degree of balance between the "this" and the "that," between the hard and the soft, between the "yes" and the "no," the firm and the yielding, the familiar and the novel, the things we do to protect ourselves and the things we do to welcome life.

Finding one's centerpoint doesn't mean giving up parts of ourselves, it means discovering new possibilities within us. It means exploring "the other side of the continuum" to get unstuck from the limiting beliefs and behaviors that have kept us in distress. It means finding balance. And with balance comes greater ease, peace, and freedom.

While the idea of the centerpoint doesn't give us a way to measure personal growth, it gives us a way to imagine it. Personal growth becomes a matter of opening up to greater possibilities, learning, being more flexible, having better access to your own inner resources, and giving up the fight to be someone you're not. By its very nature, the centerpoint is the place inside ourselves of greatest self-acceptance, greatest empowerment, greatest authenticity, and least conflict.

There is no "right" way to be in this positive model of personal growth and healing. Balance is the goal, not any particular kind of structure, prescription or creed (unless you want to consider "valuing balance" as some kind of dogma). Water seeks its own level, nature reclaims itself, and a human being, freed from the tyranny of what's familiar, will do the same.

Exploration of our "symptoms" with an attitude of curiosity will, in time, provide the insight we need to make whatever changes we need to make to achieve better balance. This is one of the greatest gifts we get from the unconscious, particularly as it expresses itself through our bodies. Within every tension is the seeds of its own relaxation (or something like that). We just need to show up, pay attention, and follow that inner wisdom to wherever it may lead. Will it lead us to write that letter we've needed to write? To assert ourselves in a way we never have before? To start meditating? To remember and tell the story of our sexual abuse? To listen more than we speak? To allow ourselves to be touched? To let someone see something in ourselves we've never shown anyone before? The possibilities are endless.

The idea that balance is central to health and wellness isn't new. We've been hearing about the benefits of a "balanced diet" for years. Many things in life are known to require balance. Riding a bicycle. Managing a checkbook. Weighing yourself at the doctor's office. Balance isn't just important when you're doing things like that. It isn't just important when you're walking a tightrope. It's important all the time.

What's special about balance in psychological health and wellness is that it's not merely something to maintain the status quo. Balance is important to bicycle riding because it keeps us upright. Balancing our checkbook keeps us out of debt. But balance in our psychology does more than just help us to avoid problems. Balance helps to keep us at peace, keeps us growing and learning, helps to keep us engaged, and makes it easier to regain our equilibrium and recover at those times in life when, despite our best efforts, we do get overwhelmed.

Finding the centerpoint requires us to pay attention and to tell the truth to ourselves (and to those who might help us and who matter to us) but it doesn't require tremendous discipline or genius. You don't have to go off to Nepal and spend seven years in silent retreat at the top of a mountain. The centerpoint is already there, within you. We don't have to create it, we just have to find it. It's not like learning how to play the sitar or interpret the kabbalah. The fundamentals are already there. You've already got the antibodies. Every one of us who needs to get more comfortable with his angry feelings to find greater balance has gotten angry before. Every one of us has cried, shouted, withdrawn, pushed back, asked, rejected, accepted, fought, and engaged in every kind of experience that might be necessary to restore balance to his system. No new vocabulary needs to be learned. Finding your centerpoint and restoring balance is a matter of re-capturing what's been lost or forgotten much more than it's about creating something new.

Admittedly, this is more philosophy than science. This new positive psychology is not designed to fit into the worldview of the pharmacomedinsurance complex. Getting unstuck is about breaking free of old patterns and restoring balance to help unlock human potential, reduce suffering, and increase wellness. It's not about treating illness. It relies on awareness and insight more than on algorithmic logic. But since when has life followed a logical course? Human experience can only be understood phenomenologically, if it can be understood at all.

We certainly can't measure personal growth because human experience exists in far more than two dimensions.

Balance can't be defined in conventional terms because it is about far more than a lack of typically recognized symptoms or traits. Some aspects of life can be measured. A body can be understood in terms of height and weight and a variety of other observable, quantifiable criteria. Psychological tests can help us make predictions about how a person might behave in this situation, or that. But the quality of a life, a person's experience of life, can't really be measured. It can only be described. And that takes getting unstuck out of the realm of mainstream therapy and into something much more, dare I say...cosmic?

Notwithstanding the lack of measurable criteria, and orbiting back down to earth, getting unstuck, finding your centerpoint, and restoring balance to your life helps people to feel, and function, better. They feel more empowered. They're more engaged, more authentically themselves. They're more focused in the present and more at peace.

Getting unstuck isn't a cure for depression or insomnia. It's never going to be FDA approved. There's never going to be a medication that will even so much as promise to help you get unstuck. But getting unstuck will make more effective whatever methods you do apply to solve your problems because it will help to free you from the stasis that helped to cause those problems in the first place. And your sense of aliveness will be enhanced, which is what personal growth is all about.

8

Finding the Centerpoint

IMAGINE THAT YOU'RE about to take a shower or bath. The first thing you do is turn on the water and seek a comfortable mix of hot and cold. Unless you're looking to shock yourself, you won't begin to bathe until the water's at a comfortable temperature. What's "too hot" to one might be "not hot enough" to another. We each have our own sense of what it means to feel comfortable and at ease. We each define our centerpoint in our own way.

So it is with most things. Each of us has his own quiet, peaceful place inside himself, where things are "just right." It's not necessarily in a fixed point in space and time, but the feeling of equanimity we associate with this place serves as a kind of touchstone. It's the place inside ourselves to which we want to return and then remain for as long as possible.

Each of us has a unique perspective. I think that the centerpoint may have already been described in numerous other languages and traditions. I can't say that the center-point means something different from what others may have already described in different terms. All of which goes to show that describing the centerpoint isn't easy.

What may distinguish the concept of the centerpoint from other efforts is that I think of the centerpoint as a bioenergetic reality, not just as a psychological construct. The centerpoint is a function of the mind/body relationship and that relation-ship is fundamentally organized around the management of energy. And by "energy" I mean prana and orgone and ch'i and elan vital and odyllic force. And I might mean atmospheric free-floating electrons, too. I'm not sure. Whatever that life-force really is. However you want to think about it. I'm just going to refer to it as "energy" and when I do that it will really be a reference to "bioenergy," which is a cumbersome word I want to try to avoid.

Since I've felt energetic streamings through my body, had positive experiences in an orgone accumulator, felt intense elec-tric-like sensations in acupuncture, and full-body orgasms, I know that there's something that moves through us that has some con-nection to positive emotion, joy, pleasure, freedom, and healing that is best understood as energy. And I'll leave it at that.

In any case, the centerpoint is something more than you could describe with just blood work and a personality test. The centerpoint is more than a sum of mind+body. It's also highly subjective. As with a person's pain level, only the person, him-self, really knows what he feels.

No matter the language or concepts or metaphors you would use to define or describe your centerpoint, there are a few things about it that would appear to me to be universally true:

- When you're there, you feel fully alive, energized

- and ready for action, but content just to be

- When you're there, you're fully present

- When you're there, your breathing is easy and unconstrained

- When you're there, you are at peace

Most, if not all, of us have had such moments in our lives. We know what the centerpoint feels like, even if we might never have spent much time thinking about it or trying to put the experience into words. Now, imagine spending more than a moment in that peaceful, balanced place. Imagine remaining there for an extended period of time. Imagine it's not just when you're bathing in that perfectly warm water or lounging at your favorite beach or curled up in the loving arms of your beloved. What might that feel like?

Some might be inclined to say it would feel like "heaven on earth." No apologies for going cosmic. After all, what could possibly be better than "heaven on earth?" More heaven on earth? (ok, for that, I will apologize.)

Years ago, I learned something about heaven that I'll never forget. I'd attended a workshop with Dr. Stan Grof on spiritual psychology in which we explored the many religious and spiritual traditions in which the death/rebirth motif plays a central role. The story of the crucifixion, then rebirth, of Jesus is really just one of many such stories. Stan's brilliant insight, the one that has stayed with me over these many years, is that the universality of the death/rebirth motif suggests that the story should never be taken literally. It is not really about dying and getting reincarnated. What the motif portrays is man experiencing the death of his suffering self and his rebirth as a spiritual being. "Heaven" is not a place we go to when we die. Rather, it's a place we go to when we find greater peace within ourselves. Now, I think we might all be better off were this to become the conventional wisdom. But I digress...

Whatever we are to call this realm of living-most-of-the-time at our centerpoint, the important thing is it's a reachable destination. Anyone can get there. And you absolutely don't need to die first!!! What you do need is a willingness to be honest with yourself, a desire to get unstuck from old patterns that are making you suffer, and a willingness to do some work along the way. It might also pay to bring along your sense of humor, because nothing is guaranteed and success doesn't mean flawlessness. Hell, I'm writing a book on how to find heaven on earth and I had a terrible day, yesterday! (Honestly, no, but I hope you get my point. Let me just say that of all the things in life I'm grateful for, laughter is near the top of the list, maybe because I so often find myself needing to find the humor in things).

Who knows if it's possible to live one's life at the centerpoint? Like I've said, this is not science, per se, and we're talking about something that's impossible to measure. But does that matter? There are any number of things to be wary of in this life and, frankly, anyone promising you nirvana is one of those things to be wary of. Getting unstuck so that you can live more of your life in an enhanced sense of aliveness with a greater sense of peace is what this book is about, not about how to find God (although some people might argue that they're the same thing...that's their business).

In any case, the journey to your centerpoint begins with an honest inventory of your bioenergetic status. To do this, you need to understand a basic bioenergetic principle: Your mind/body organizes itself around its need to manage energy.

Energy moves through us and finds its expression in both mind and body. In the former, energy is transformed into thought and creativity. In the latter, it's transformed into movement. What we refer to as emotion represents the unified experience of mind/body: our minds interpret the movement of energy through our bodies as "feeling." Efforts to limit, or otherwise manipulate, feeling result in the development of chronic bioenergetic tensions affecting both mind and body. To some extent, chronic bioenergetic tensions may be necessary, as they help to preserve "order," both internally and in terms of society as a whole. But chronic bioenergetic tensions which leave us significantly out of balance are destructive, as they can impair our capacity to feel, to learn, to love, to heal, and to grow.

The mind/body is, in other words, an energetic system. Like any energetic system, it takes in energy, utilizes it, then discharges it. Imbalances show up as "undercharge" or "overcharge," which are experiential, if not quantifiable, states of being. Both conditions are indicative of musculoskeletal and/or mental rigidity that I call being "stuck." The centerpoint refers to a place of energetic balance within the mind/body. While the centerpoint may not be a measurable phenomenon, it is experienced as a place of balance, or greater balance, wherein a person feels at peace, fully alive, and neither under- nor overcharged.

Bioenergetic rigidities develop at the "charge" or "discharge" points of the charge → activation → discharge → relaxation cycle. The qualities of "activation" and of "relaxation" are directly proportional to the freedom of "charge" and "discharge." Unimpeded "charging" of the system results in the greatest potential for "activation" and unimpeded "discharging" allows for the greatest degree of "relaxation." Rigidification of the system interferes with the energetic system and creates imbalance. Getting "unstuck" is like undergoing a "de-rigidification" of the energetic system. The centerpoint is the place of maximum de-rigidification.

Each person's energetic story is unique. How, when, and why we develop our particular pattern of rigidity, of being stuck, is a reflection of our idiosyncratic experiences. And it would be wrong to suggest that one pattern is "better" than another. We develop the patterns we develop because: 1) we had to do something to cope with the circumstances we faced; and 2) we did what we could. None of us learned that everything about who we are is good. We all learned that something(s) about who we are, what we feel, what we enjoy, or how we might choose to express ourselves is not acceptable. So, we made our bioenergetic adjustments. Less of this and none of that.

Not surprisingly, the bioenergetic patterns we've developed are often very much like those of our parents. Might this be part of our genetic endowment? It's certainly possible. It is common to speak of character traits like "temper" and "stubbornness" and "sense of humor" as being similar to that of one's mother or father, so why not our bioenergetic structure? We most certainly do inherit all kinds of tendencies, so it wouldn't make sense to exclude from that list our bioenergetic tendencies, would it? And it is undeniably so that most people marry someone whose emotional style is "familiar" to them (essentially, someone who is "just like the girl who married dear old dad," or mom). That we tend to raise our children similarly to the ways in which we, ourselves, were raised, follows from this. I'll leave the "nature or nurture" question for others to debate. I'd say, "it's both." Yin and yang. Yang and yin. It's important, again, to remember that we need to approach such matters with curiosity, not with judgment. Our bioenergetic patterns developed out of need, not out of stupidity. We all needed to cope and we did the best we could.

Psychological labels can be useful, but they can also be destructive. I love psychology and proudly identify myself with the field. But it is imperfect science. For example, intelligence tests, one of the great contributions to human knowledge developed by psychologists, are useful, but limited. Everyone knows about "IQ" and understands that higher numbers are associated with "higher intelligence." But "IQ" doesn't take into account, at all, a person's creativity or the strength of their aspiration or drive. "IQ" means something, for sure, but it isn't a good predictor of success, however you might want to measure that. People with high IQ scores often do poorly in school and fail in their personal relationships. People with average IQ scores often do well in their businesses and have happy marriages. Years ago, "Esquire" magazine profiled a young man who'd reportedly scored the highest in his generation on a commonly used intelligence test. He was, in other words, "the smartest guy in the room." Any and every room, that is. He'd dropped out of college and was working as a bartender. Not as a nuclear physicist. Judgment would lead one to think of him as a "disappointment." After all, he's "just a bartender and you don't need an IQ of 173 to be a bartender." But maybe he's content. Maybe he'd rather be a happy bartender than a miserable research scientist. I hope he doesn't care what anyone else thinks. And how many people have been hurt by being labelled as "dumb" in school because they struggled with reading or did poorly on standardized achievement tests? You might not find many Nobel prize winners who are dyslexic or who were poor at math, but you'd certainly find plenty of CEOs, lawyers, great artists, and good parents who were. Many people who might've been successful in their lives were crippled by getting labeled negatively when they were young. There's no psychological test that measures "resilience," and that might be as important a trait to personal success as any.

Professional biases and labelling aside, we all need to approach the work of personal growth with curiosity rather than judgment. After all, judgment has had a lot to do with how we all got stuck in the first place. The feelings we've come to deny and reject are never "wrong" or "bad" in and of themselves. Sadness, anger, sensitivity, tenderness, stubbornness—all of them may serve a useful, life-affirming function if we embrace them as part of who we are rather than as pathology, as disease, as defects. Personal growth is about expanding our sense of who we are and what we might experience. It can never be about de-valuing ourselves—-or any part of ourselves. Judgment often leads to de-valuation.

Curiosity leads to compassion. Curiosity allows for deeper understanding. Curiosity is, essentially, about love. It is about accepting reality rather than fighting with it. It is, for example, about acknowledging your anger and questioning its function in your life rather than holding onto the idea that "anger is bad." It is about accepting your sensitivity rather than holding onto the idea that "sensitivity makes a person weak." Curiosity is about loving yourself rather than fearing yourself, i.e. being open to self-discovery rather than being scared of what you might find.

An honest inventory must begin with curiosity. I say this because, let's face it, we're all inclined to be judgmental—especially about ourselves—-and maybe, even, a little dishonest.

We don't like to admit our weaknesses, fears, or blindspots. We all expect judgment from others "if they only knew" because we are judgmental, ourselves.

Self-judgment feeds our suffering. Self-judgment is usually yet another indication of being "stuck" because those self-judgments reflect negative beliefs we learned in childhood and have held onto throughout our lives—despite the damage they've done. Letting go of, or moving past, self-judgment and cultivating an attitude of curiosity is as simple as deciding that you're tired of suffering and want to take the leap into wellness. Not necessarily easy, but it is simple.

The biggest impediment to letting go of judgment is your ego.

Ego can be defined in many ways, but I think of it as the "social self," the personality we present to the world. The ego doesn't reflect well the person who we really are. Most of the time, at least, it reflects the person whom we want others to see, and that is different from the person who we really are. The ego is a direct result of our judgments and fears. If we expect condemnation for being insecure, we present an arrogant self to the world. That's ego. If we need to have people think of us as infallible, we blame others for our mistakes. That's ego. It wouldn't be unreasonable to think of the ego as the "pretend self." And, as Kurt Vonnegut once wrote, "we must be careful about what we pretend to be." Pretension might help in some realms of life, but it won't help you get unstuck.

The ego won't help you get unstuck because the stuck self is the ego. Yes, that is another way of understanding things. The stuck self—your ego— is the self you've been presenting to the world. And—here's the kicker— despite all your suffering, your ego is perfectly content. Your ego has no incentive to change. Your ego has no interest in growth or healing. Your ego tries to control things so that it can maintain its own existence. Your ego doesn't suffer. You may suffer, but your ego doesn't. The ego is not alive; it has no feelings to get hurt. So you can't rely on your ego to help get you unstuck. You've got to rely on something real. Your mind/body. Your true self. Your soul. That part of you that does feel, that can love, that is tired of suffering and welcomes change. That's the part of you willing to take an honest look at your bioenergetic status, recognize the truth, and approach that truth with curiosity.

I don't know if it's possible to let go of one's ego completely. I don't even know if it's necessary. There are religious practices that purport to help people dissolve their egos. But this book is not about any kind of religious practice. What I do think is possible, and necessary, is to loosen the grip of the ego. Spending less time being "ego-driven" is important to personal growth because, as I've said, the ego resists change.

Because the ego is the stuck self, it is bound up in our mind/body tensions. Anything we do to relax those tensions, even for just a moment, helps to loosen the ego's grip. When I do group sessions, I'll often begin with a simple exercise to help people relax, so that they will be more open to the feelings and insights that might come from the group process:

Find a comfortable place to sit. Close your eyes. Notice your breath.

How does your breathing feel? Be aware of any tensions that may be getting in the way...Now begin to breathe in through your nose and out through your mouth. Let your jaw relax so that nothing blocks the outflow. Now imagine that, beginning at the area of your nose and mouth, there is a flexible hollow tube that extends all the way down through your throat and chest into your belly. Each time you inhale now, you draw your breath all the way down into your belly and you can feel it fill with each inhalation, then flatten again when you exhale. After each exhalation, now, silently, to yourself, say the word "relax." Relax. Relax...

The centerpoint is a place of balance inside each one of us. It is a place of relative equivalence of charge and discharge which allows for the maximum pulsation of our bioenergetic system. The journey to the centerpoint begins with an honest appraisal of your current bioenergetic status, so that you can understand your imbalances and what you must do to recalibrate your system.

Some bodies are hard, taught, muscled. Others are softer and seem more yielding. Some carry themselves with a "military bearing," i.e. chest out, shoulders back, stomach in, etc. Some carry themselves with more slumped shoulders. Some eyes are wide open; others peer sharply out from under a furrowed brow. Some of us are all too happy to welcome others into our private world of feelings while others keep their emotional distance. Some of us are happy to do nothing much at all while others can't ever seem to slow down. None of these traits is bad. None of these traits is good. Each makes sense energetically and says something about the energetic character of a person.

To find your centerpoint, which is your point of greater balance, you need to understand how your system is currently out of balance, and how you've been using your body and mind to maintain your energetic status quo. Then, using that centerpoint as a reference, you get engaged in an ongoing process of personal growth that helps to get you, and keep you, unstuck.

9

The Bioenergetic Map

LIKE ANY OTHER energetic system, the mind/body gets charged, activated, then discharges. As it charges, it fills, and as it fills its internal tension increases. As it discharges, it empties, and as it empties, it relaxes. This cycle of contraction and expansion is the fundamental pulsation in all living beings and distinguishes the living from the non-living. Death could fairly be described as the moment when pulsation stops.

Numerous physical activities within the human body can be understood as pulsation, but especially the contraction and expansion of the lungs— and their associated musculoskeletal structures—and the beating of the heart. Less obvious, but no less important, are the pulsations of mind, primarily found in the rhythms of social contact and withdrawal and the cadences of thought and expression. Every one of these pulsations represents the taking in of energy, the processing or utilization of that energy, and its discharge.

As with any energetic system, some type of balance must be maintained to ensure that the system functions adequately and doesn't deteriorate or explode. In mechanical systems, the inflow and outflow of energy can, typically, be easily regulated. Step down on the gas pedal, the engine burns up more fuel and the car accelerates. Let up on the gas pedal and the opposite occurs. With mechanical systems and more conventional sources of energy, balance is straightforward, measurable, and predictable. In living systems, and in the realm of the more subtle lifeforce to which we've been referring, maintaining balance is a more complex matter.

The human being is, unlike a car or a vacuum cleaner, more than the sum of his parts. People are multidimensional and, while certain physical dimensions, such as height, weight, heart rate, and caloric consumption are quantifiable, other dimensions, especially those which are non-physical, resist mathematical definition. The ways in which the mind/body strives to maintain energetic balance are challenging to define and impossible to measure. As Alfred Korzybski famously said, "the map is not the territory." The best we can hope for, in trying to understand the matter of bioenergetic balance in the mind/body, is a map that helps to describe the territory but refrains from trying to define it.

Certainly, every living person maintains some degree of energetic balance. People do not implode and explode spontaneously, which is what would happen were the mind/body to be totally energetically overwhelmed. Every one of us "holds it together" well enough, at least, to keep breathing, keep our skeletons intact, and to maintain some sense of individual identity. Even if we "fall apart," we don't do so completely.

Because "perfect energetic balance" may be more of a theoretical construct than an achievable reality, it may be useful to think of a "compensatory" energetic system in which an imbalance in one aspect is matched by an inverse imbalance elsewhere. Thinking about such a compensatory system puts me in mind of Ida Rolf, whose technique of "structural integration" sought to help re-align a body around its center of gravity. Rolf believed that the body worked most efficiently when it is so aligned. The "Rolfer" drops an imaginary plumb line through his client's body which allows for him to visualize all the ways in which the bends and twists on one side of the line get compensated for by corresponding bends and twists on the other side that allow even for the very "misaligned" client to continue to defy gravitational force and keep walking upright, though perhaps without ease and grace.

"Bioenergetic character" refers to the things that people do to hold their energetic systems together. This would include not just the business of coping with gravity, but also coping with the demands of both our inner world and our outer, social lives. As we've already seen, people tend towards different degrees of "boundedness," with greater boundedness associated with greater containment of energetic charge. The "underbounded" character tends towards a lack of energy while the "overbounded" character tends to accumulate too much.

"Boundedness" is a function of armoring, which naturally develops as chronic musculoskeletal tensions and/or psychological defenses designed to limit our energetic experience. Overboundedness and underboundedness can lead to problems, but energetic boundaries are essential to survival as they serve a need to limit experience at times when experience would otherwise be overwhelming. Boundaries help us to adjust to the society all around us, they help to keep us safe, they help us to focus, and they help us cope with the various traumas, injuries, and stressful circumstances we all must face.

A map of energetic character that I've found to be useful looks like this:

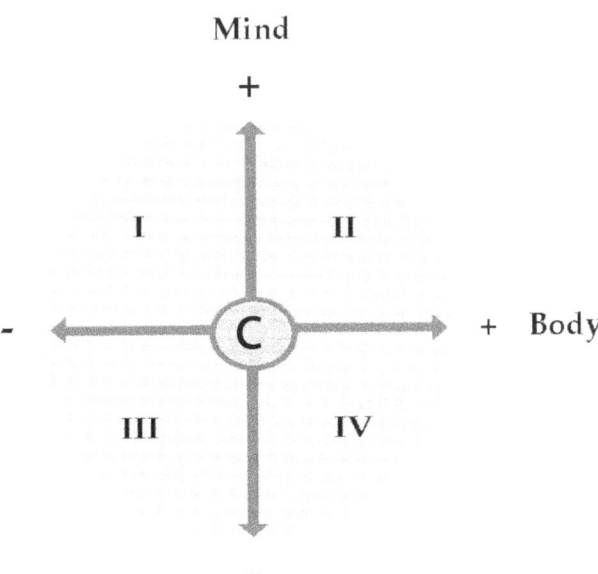

While this simple, two-dimensional schema may not be more than a finger pointing to a multidimensional moon, it can help, at the very least, to put the unknowable and indescribable into some kind of usable form.

What it depicts is an interrelated, interactive mind/body system organized around the function of managing energy. Both "mind" and "body" are viewed as interrelated energetic structures which can be undercharged or overcharged. The centerpoint is placed in the middle, but not at the mathematical center, which is intended to reflect its subjective and mutable nature.

What you can see from this map right away is that bioenergetic character is always a reflection of mind and body and that the energetic relationship between the two may be either complementary or parallel. In other words, an "overbounded" mind can be paired with an "underbounded" body, or vice versa; alternatively, one can find a mind/body system in which both aspects are either over- or underbounded. This allows for some categorization of energetic character while, at the same time, acknowledging the nearly limitless subtle differences we may find as we look into the ways in which people strive to maintain energetic balance.

The mind/body, as I'm describing it here, functions like an hydraulic system. Each mind/body is capable of just so much energetic capacity and the maintenance of balance is a matter of relating input and output. Energetic capacity might change over time, but not the need for balance. Overcharge in one aspect gets balanced by undercharge in the other aspect and vice versa. Yin and yang. Yang and yin. Mind/body systems that function in parallel tend to be far more out of balance than those which are complementary.

The map also provides a visual guide to the work of getting unstuck. Getting unstuck from old patterns always involves the same basic thing: movement toward the centerpoint. No matter where you might find yourself on the map, the journey towards the centerpoint represents the direction of greater pulsation, greater freedom, greater personal growth, greater balance.

Looking at the map, there are, essentially, four core bioenergetic character types. While the two complementary types (I and IV) tend to be more balanced than the systems in parallel (II and III), each reflects the best efforts a person has made to cope and survive. Each reflects an individual's emotional history, i.e. how loved and safe he felt growing up and what kinds of expectations he has of the world around him. Each type reflects particular ways of being stuck and unique challenges to the work of getting unstuck. Each type is reflective of the kinds and quality of the boundaries we've established to meet the requirements of managing energy and the psychological and physical structures we've developed as a result. Those psychological and physical structures are apparent in the way we look and in the way we act.

Each of us is unique in terms of our appearance and our behavior. But we all, no matter our personal history or genetic endowment, want to feel like we're in charge of our own lives, that we've got a sense of our own identity and personal power. That's universal. Boundaries, which are both psychological and physical in nature, help us to achieve this sense of sovereignty by establishing something that feels like a "personal space." Inside of that space is "me" and outside of that space lies everything and everybody else. As long as my sense of that personal space is clear, my sovereignty is intact. I'm empowered. I'm in charge of the territory I call "me" and you're not. When our sense of that personal space is unclear, or insufficiently developed, our sovereignty is easily threatened. We are disempowered. And, in that state, we are anxious and insecure. Personal sovereignty—the sense of being in charge of our own lives—- isn't just given to us and can't just be taken for granted. In fact, it needs to be cultivated. When we're faced with challenges or threats, it needs to be defended.

When other people challenge our personal space in some way and threaten our sense of feeling "in charge," we defend ourselves with anger. That's what anger is all about: the emotion that's triggered by threats to our sense of self-governance. In the best circumstances, we can channel and express such angry feeling in an appropriate way and, in doing so, defend and preserve our sense of "self." This is why people who can't fully embrace their anger tend to struggle with their identity and their sense of empowerment. Ideally, the need to defend and preserve gets triggered only by real threats (rather than fantasy). Absent a genuine challenge or threat, we're calm and at peace. Unfortunately, we're not always calm and at peace and the challenges and threats we face don't always come from other people. They often come from within.

If energy is allowed to move too freely through a body, let's say because of underdeveloped muscular armoring, emotions can run wild. A well-functioning person does have to be in touch with emotions and experience them fully. But he also needs to be able to turn off the emotional spigot, as well. Work needs to get done. Responsibilities need to be kept. Communications need to be clear. We need to be able to let go and let in and use adequate discernment between the two. We need to cope emotionally with our world while not making it too difficult for the world to cope with us. Our personal space needs not just to be adequately defended but also well-nurtured and well-organized. Emotions and impulses running amok would make all that impossible. This is the positive function of the armoring. Too much of it might get in the way, but too little and our lives turn into chaos.

So maintaining bioenergetic balance, which is, for our purposes here, equally thought of as psychological balance, or even physical balance, is essential to our well-being. If we wind up allowing too much energy to move through us, we feel too much and our lives—our personal spaces— become chaotic. If we don't allow energy to move freely enough through us, our lives become stale.

Maintaining energetic balance involves our minds and our bodies, both of which are energetic entities that utilize energy to function and work together to maintain some overall balance of the system. Bodies feel and move. Minds think and create. The relative energetic interplay between mind and body is what is reflected in the idea of bioenergetic character.

Mind and body work together to manage the energy that moves through the mind/body.

Efforts to limit, channel, and balance the input/output of the mind/body result in both musculoskeletal and psychological patterning. We see this patterning in the ways people hold their bodies. Some stand upright, the tops of their heads parallel to the ground, their legs firm. Others are sway-backed, longer over the lengths of their torsos, shoulders retracted, hips forward, hyperextended through their knees. Others carry themselves more rigidly, with little movement through their upper bodies, intensity in their eyes, their chests thrust forward. People also develop psychological patterns of behavior to manage energy. Some withdraw into themselves to try to avoid absorbing too much energy from the world around them, while others are able to put up a virtual "keep out" sign. Some give in easily while others remain defiant.

It would be impossible to describe in detail all the ways in which minds and bodies develop in their efforts to manage energy. There are an infinite number of patterns, combinations, and permutations. While you might look at the two axes of the bioenergetic map and see two long continuums, what separates one end of the pole from the other is really a very short distance. We are all imperfectly balanced. We all have both undercharged and overcharged aspects of ourselves, fears, and places where we are unhealed. We are all stuck in some ways. And we all have to cope with the fundamental paradox of our bioenergetic life: that armoring gets in our way but is also essential to our well-being. Armoring tends to keep all of us stuck, but we might all be gelatinous energized blobs of inchoate flesh, bone, and brain without it. Getting unstuck doesn't involve getting rid of armor, but rather, becoming more aware of it and loosening it up so we can get back on a life path of personal growth instead of static suffering.

In other words, even while one bioenergetic type might seem more balanced, or healthier, than another, none is perfect. None is unstuck. None is devoid of challenges. None is devoid of strengths. None can't learn to function better. All need to be approached with curiosity, rather than judgment. Our concern here is with what these various bioenergetic types can help us learn about ourselves—and, for therapists, about the people with whom they work—and about what it will take to get unstuck from old patterns and onto a path of personal growth.

10

Finding Your Energetic Type

IF I EAT a grapefruit, I consume 85 calories, or so. And if after eating the grapefruit, I go out for a short walk and that walk burns up 84 calories, my body is going to store 1 calorie, or so, in reserve. We can measure these things. Balancing a diet can be done with a scale and a calculator.

Not so with bioenergetics. When we're talking about subtle energy, we enter into the realm of the mysterious, the immeasurable, maybe even the numinous. We can't calculate bioenergetic balance. We can't measure how stuck we are. We can only feel it.

But we can feel it. When we're stuck, we don't feel well. We lack vitality and, maybe, even feel depressed. We feel stressed, insecure, anxious. We don't feel fully alive, fully present, fully engaged. We feel burdened, harried, conflicted. We may be "OK," but we're not good. Or, perhaps more accurately, we're not as good as we'd like to be.

When we're unstuck, we're at peace. When we're unstuck, there's no lingering tension. No anxiety. The voice inside us is quiet. Everything might not be perfect, but all is well. When we're unstuck, our mind/body vibrates at the frequency of "ahhhh." Or, even better, at the frequency of "Om."

Funny thing about "Om." A dear friend of mine explained it to me once. There's three sounds people make to express the feeling of pleasure. No matter where you go or what language is being spoken, people say either "aah" or "oh" or "mmm" to express their pleasure. Put the three together— "aah" +

"oh" + "mmm"——and what do you get?

"Om." The universal sound of pleasure. The sound the mind/body makes when it's unstuck.

Some might think you have to practice intensive meditation to get to that place of pleasure. Or renounce all of your worldly possessions. Or pray three times each day. Or read the Egyptian Book of the Dead, the Upanishads, and the collected works of Gurdjieff whilst sitting in a full lotus position on a fourteen day fast. But you don't. Nothing against such practices, of course. But the work of getting unstuck doesn't involve quite that level of discipline, dedication, and devotion. Getting unstuck requires only awareness, some courage, and a willingness to try new things.

That awareness begins with an honest assessment of your bioenergetic type because you need to understand how you've been managing your energy before you can start managing your energy differently. Your centerpoint is, after all, not just a point of greater energetic balance, but also a destination on a map. You need to know where you are on the map if you're going to take the proper route to your destination.

"Overbounded" is always suggestive of strong armor and a higher energetic charge. An overbounded entity tends to store, or hold in, its energy and tends to resist more than it yields. Since the mind is the aspect of our bioenergetic system we use to make social contact, the overbounded mind is one that tends to resist intimacy and the sharing of feelings. The overbounded mind is, in the classic sense, "defensive." By "defensive" is meant that a person with an overbounded mind is guarded, perhaps no more than sufficiently so, but guarded, nonetheless. The psychological boundaries of the person with an overbounded mind are firm. But in the highly overbounded person (imagine someone at the north end of the "mind" axis), the boundaries can border on the impenetrable.

The overbounded mind is, if anything, controlled. It is not prone to making impulsive choices or blatant, dramatic expressions of emotion. It keeps its energy contained. The overbounded mind is deliberative, rational, cautious to a fault. The strong psychological boundaries of the person with an overbounded mind can serve him well. He can limit energetic input when he needs to. He can avoid getting overwhelmed by the energy of other people's thoughts and feelings, especially when that energy is disturbing or toxic. He can keep himself psychologically safe.

What he can't do so well, however, is receive new experience. The psychologically overbounded mind is not a receptive mind. It doesn't welcome what's new quite so easily and this can really limit new learning. The psychologically overbounded person may do a good job of keeping himself safe but being stuck in safety mode tends to keep his life going around in a circle. Rather than learning, healing, growing, he stagnates.

Tunnel vision and stubbornness, which are manifestations of psychological overboundedness, can be strengths. They can give a person the capability of filtering out the extraneous and staying "on task" no matter the circumstances. But they can also render a person incapable of flexibility and of making necessary adjustments when he needs to. It is one thing to be able to hold firm to one's beliefs or vision; it is something else entirely to hold firm to one's beliefs or vision even after you've been presented with evidence that you're heading in the wrong direction.

Mental armor develops, as all armor does, for a complex of reasons. The mental armor that we need to help us channel the energy of our thoughts into purposeful, meaningful action is critical to living a productive life and to the competency fundamental to personal growth. A basic capacity to defend ourselves against unwanted, unwelcome people and ideas is essential. We need to be able to keep out of our personal space the energy of others we find disturbing or toxic. Psychological defenses—our social boundaries—are a reflection of our mental armor.

What we might think of as "hyper-defensiveness" is an indication not of well-developed mental armor but of excessive overboundedness. The person possessed of excessive over-bounded, overcharged mental armor—the "hyper-defensive" person— doesn't just defend himself from hurt. He's stuck in an old pattern of defending himself from becoming en-meshed. Fear is what maintains the excessively overbounded mind, not love and trust. To the extent a person's history is marked by enmeshment trauma, his psychological armoring is hardened.

Hardened armor loses its flexibility and adaptability. The "hyper-defensive" person isn't taking good care of himself in the present moment. He's trying to protect himself from something, or someone, in his past and cope with an energetic wound that's never been healed. Think back for a moment to Terry...

It is a good thing, a strength, to be clear about one's needs and beliefs, likes and dislikes, and to be able to ward off those people and things we find uninteresting, disagreeable, or tox-ic. It is not such a good thing to be so defensive that we are broadly dismissive, chronically angry, combative, and toxic to others.

Psychological underboundedness, on the other hand, is suggestive of less well-developed armoring and lower ener-getic charge. Energy doesn't get contained here; it gets easily, and sometimes indiscriminately, discharged. Lack of mental— or psychological—boundedness often leads to a person not being able to control himself, even when he needs to. Such losses of control can manifest in a number of ways, but es-pecially as emotional outbursts and/or an inability to regain one's emotional composure under stress. The lack of capacity for containment and control is also often associated with problems focusing, concentrating, managing time, and completing tasks.

If defensiveness is a hallmark of a psychologically overbounded person, sensitivity and vulnerability are what distinguish the psychologically underbounded. While the psychologically overbounded person resists intimacy and, if anything, tends to "live in his head," the sensitivity, openness, and natural empathy of the psychologically underbounded person gives them a great capacity to share their thoughts and feelings freely and develop intimacy. This is, of course, a real strength in terms of relationship. But, as with the seriously overbounded individual, those strengths in the seriously underbounded individual (imagine the south pole of the "mind" axis) can, on the flip side, lead to problems. A seriously underbounded individual may develop intimacy too quickly, sometimes even before establishing the safety and viability of the relationship. In other words, the seriously psychologically underbounded person might tend to be receptive to the energy of another too quickly and with inadequate discernment. Thus, the attachments he makes can be volatile and unstable, often marked by dramatic shifts in mood and tenor.

What underlies the relative lack of armoring in the psychologically underbounded person, more than anything else, and what tends to keep them stuck, is pervasive fear of abandonment. This fear has its historical antecedent in parental instability. While the parent(s) of the psychologically overbounded were too demanding, too intrusive, too over-bearing, the parent(s) of the psychologically underbounded were not consistently present enough and were unstable. This created a situation wherein the child became funda-mentally insecure and learned to get, and cling to, love and nurturance whenever, and from whomever, it was available, whether, or not, that love was marked by other indications of safety and wholesomeness. This is why, so often, a psychologi-cally underbounded person accumulates a personal history of relationships tainted by instability, volatility, and abuse. The psychologically underbounded person lacks the armoring needed to make deliberative choices about intimate matters and often mistakes limerence for true love. Making connec-tions comes easily to the psychologically underbounded, but their emotional intensity and relative lack of capacity to con-tain their impulses and feelings can make their social judgment poor and their relationships unstable.

That all said, none of us is purely this or purely that. The map is not the territory. Yin and yang. Yang and Yin. We are all overbounded. And underbounded. It's only a matter of degree that distinguishes one of us from another energetically. Each of us lies somewhere along the same axes, tied together by our common need to find energetic balance, separated only by the ways in which we choose to do it. Try to approach the question of where you lie on the continuum with curiosity rather than judgment.

Physical armor gives us the capacity to contain and chan-nel energy, functions which are essential to the empowerment needed for personal growth. If we can't physically bind energy adequately, we wind up not just undercharged but also disempowered. And if we can't hold back emotions when we need to hold them back, our lives become chaotic. On the other hand, if we can't surrender to our feelings when the moment calls for it, our emotional life is deadened, our wounds can't heal, and our capacity for sexual and sensual pleasure is blunted. Such is the complex function of armoring: it doth giveth and taketh away.

Unlike the psychological armoring, which can only be implied from observing behavior, the physical armoring provides some direct evidence of its existence in the physical form of our bodies, in our patterns of muscular development, and in how we breathe and carry ourselves. The bodies of underbounded and overbounded people don't just manage energy differently; they look and move differently, too.

I'm speaking especially of the upper torso, as that's the area most closely associated with the breathing functions. It is there, in the shape and movement of the chest and abdomen, where we find the most direct evidence of the muscular armor as it relates to the energetic charge/discharge phenomenon. Other areas of the body provide feedback about how we manage energy—our eyes, for example—but the upper torso is key to distinguishing whether a body tends generally towards overboundedness or underboundedness.

The overbounded body is, generally speaking, overcharged and expanded in the area of the chest. It's as if he, or she, is stuck on the "inhalation" stroke of breathing. High energy, but also high tension, as the musculature of the chest and its supporting apparatus through the upper back, sides, and shoulders, is chronically overcharged. This may, or may not be, associated with chronic inflammation of underlying structures but, certainly, the overcharged situation is the kind people are referring to when the talk is of "high stress" or "controlled" or, in more extreme circumstances, "ready to explode."

The diaphragm, the main muscle of breathing, is more tightly contracted in the overbounded person, which limits the depth of the person's breathing and, especially, the quality of exhalation. A tightly contracted diaphragm will limit expansion of the inhalation into the lower aspect of the lungs and will also exert tension in the mid- to lower back. This low back tension is often associated with a rearward tilt of the pelvis, at one end, and a pulling up and back of the shoulders, on the other end, resulting in a body that's longer through the front than through the back and tilted to the rear side of its center of gravity. Some of the chronic back pain problems that so many people have may be more related to this dynamic than to any other organic cause.

You might be thinking, at this point, "Yeah, but aren't such structural things as these congenital? After all, people just tend to look like their parents..."

The answer is "yes." And "no." Of course, genetics may well play a role. It would be silly to suggest otherwise. But it would be equally absurd, once you understand the energetic functions of these various musculoskeletal developments, to suggest that learning (read: nurturance) played no role. As

I've said before, most people raise their children in the same basic ways they, themselves, had been raised. So we inherit more than just genetic endowments from our parents. We also learn to deal with our emotions in similar ways. The armoring we develop may well be due to both congenital and environmental influences, but no one really knows enough to say that it's just one and not the other. Yin and yang. Yang and yin.

Armoring functions to contain and channel energy and, in the overbounded body, energy gets tightly controlled. Since we experience the movement of energy through our bodies as emotion, the overbounded individual is an emotionally controlled individual, particularly with regard to more tender feelings like sadness. In more extreme instances—think of the "eastern" point on the "body" axis—the overbounded person is incapable of either deep laughter ("belly laughs") or crying, for to do either, the diaphragm would have to swing freely and one's exhalation would have to be unblocked.

The tight, rigid musculature of the severely overbounded person gets in the way.

While there may, indeed, be some positive value in being able to tightly control one's emotions when a real need arises, chronic tightening—being stuck—can limit one's experience of life. The seriously overbounded person can't laugh fully or cry deeply. But he can't have a full and complete orgasm, either. Reich had explored this subject exhaustively in his writings about "orgastic potency."

The underbounded person carries a very different energetic dynamic. He's emotionally under-controlled, not because he isn't stuck, but because he's stuck in such a way that he's unable to contain his energy even when he needs to. Unlike his overbounded counterpart, he feels too much. His emotions flow too freely. Not being able to hold on tightly enough to his own energy, he tends to be in a chronic state of energetic depletion. If the overbounded person might be characterized as "tightly wound," the underbounded person could be called "loosely held together."

The upper torso of the underbounded person tends to be chronically contracted, as if it's stuck on the exhalation beat of the charge/discharge cycle. The underbounded character struggles not with letting go, but with taking in. This leaves him chronically undercharged. The tension in his diaphragm is, if anything, insufficient to allow for him to inhale fully, so he's always struggling to get enough energy. His problem isn't one of not enough emotion. To the contrary, he tends to feel too much and lacks the capacity to contain, or hold in, feeling even when he needs to (as, for example, when he's not in a "safe" or "appropriate" setting or when he needs to set aside his emotions for the sake of getting other business taken care of). In extreme situations—think of the westernmost point on the "body" axis—he can become almost paralyzed by his inner emotional chaos.

The frontward tilt of the underbounded body, like the rearward tilt of the overbounded body, isn't just a point of observation. It's also an indication of grounding. This is a term that gets used in a lot of different ways, but, for our purposes here, at least, refers to the relationship between the upper body and the lower body.

The more "grounded" a person, the more aligned he is around his center of gravity and, as a result of that, the steadier he is on his feet. He moves more gracefully as his connection to the ground is strongly affirmed. This steadiness of the well-grounded person is reflected both physically and psychologically in his sense of balance and in "knowing where he stands." The more "tilt," the less grounding. Problems with grounding can affect people of all energetic character types.

I want to reiterate that, in assessing your own energetic character (or in making an assessment of a client), it is important to keep in mind that, while one or the other of "overbounded" or "underbounded" might seem "better" or "healthier," there are positives and negatives all around-and that every one of us is possessed of the potential for change. Underbounded types might be prone to getting overwhelmed by their feelings and struggle to maintain focus, but their natural sensitivity and receptivity can enhance their capacity for making deep connections and acquiring new experience. Overbounded types might have a tendency to keep themselves too tightly emotionally controlled, but that same capacity for control can make them stress-hardy and undistractible. We can all—no matter our energetic character—- get unstuck from old patterns and re-orient ourselves to a life of greater vitality, healing, and growth. Moving towards the centerpoint is the key, not self-hatred or giving up who we already are. Underbounded traits are neither "good" nor "bad." Overbounded traits are, likewise, neither "good" nor "bad." Being stuck is the problem. The traits we have, the ways in which we manage energy, are a result of nature and nurture, what we were born into and learned along the way. They're not ever the result of stupidity or lack of effort.

Looking at the bioenergetic map, there are four quadrants created by the intersection of the two axes, each of which portrays a different pattern of energetic balance. The upper left quadrant represents the Type I character which trends in the direction of "overbounded mind/underbounded body." The upper right quadrant represents Type II, "overbounded body/ overbounded mind." The lower left quadrant represents Type III "underbounded body/underbounded mind" and the lower right quadrant Type IV, "overbounded body/ underbounded mind." Because these categories are broad and are meant to provide only a generalized representation of bioenergetic dynamics, each one ought to be able to find his (or her) Type.

To paraphrase Alcoholics Anonymous, taking an "honest inventory" of your psychological and physical traits is crucial here. Remember that we're looking at your energetic character, not your desirability or aptitude . This map is all about how people manage their energy, not about their moral values, sexual preferences, politics, size, race, intellectual capacity, or any one of a long list of things that make people interesting and which people tend to have judgments about. So, when you ask yourself about which energetic Type most closely aligns with the honest experience you have of yourself, do so without judgment. You manage your energy as best as your nature and nurture have allowed. We can all love. We can all grow. We can all get unstuck.

So, how are your bioenergetics? How are you really doing in body and in mind? How do you manage your energy? Ask yourself the following questions:

1. Do I tend to feel over or under-energized?

2. Do I tend to feel calm or am I prone to tension?

3. When I'm under stress, am I prone more to anger or to anxiety?

4. Do I usually feel like I can breathe freely, or do I feel like I can never get a deep enough inhalation or a full enough exhalation?

5. Do people tend to see me as overcharged or undercharged?

6. Do I generally feel in control of my emotions, especially fear and anger?

7. Do other people see me as in-control?

8. Can I fully enjoy pleasurable activity?

9. Do people find me more warm and emotional or cool and detached?

10. Am I defensive? Do others see me as defensive?

11. Do I tend to think my way through or feel my way through?

12. In which descriptions of boundedness in mind and body did I most recognize myself?

These questions provide a simple framework for finding your place on the bioenergetic map. They're not meant to be conclusive or specific. The degree of detail is up to you. You can go as deeply into your mind/body as you choose. Or, perhaps it would be better to suggest that you can go as multi- dimensionally into your mind/body as you choose. Whatever you wish. A general description of your bioenergetic status is all that's needed to begin your journey. Sometimes considering how we might be perceived by other people can help to sharpen a self-assessment, so a couple of questions refer to that.

As for the first question, about energy level, it's straightforward. How. Do. You. Feel? Since we're in the energetic realm, your self-assessment, while completely subjective, is as reliable as any. We all know whether, or not, we feel well-energized.

Question 2 asks about your general, or "resting," or "default" state of being. Calmness is associated with relaxation in the body and stillness in the mind. Tension is associated with holding back energy in the muscular armor.

Question #3 is a more direct reference to "boundedness."

Overbounded, higher energy people tend to feel and get more angry under stress. Their aggressiveness, at such times, can serve them well—so no judgment!!

Underbounded people tend to become more anxious at such moments.

With regard to breathing, most people, if asked, will say "Of course I breathe enough." That is, unless you suffer with asthma or some other kind of chronic respiratory ailment. (The bioenergetic map has nothing to say about auto-immune diseases.) This question about breathing is another totally subjective matter. Do you feel like your breathing could be more complete?

Sometimes, in doing any kind of self-assessment, it is worth trying to look at one's self from the outside, or, in other words, consider the feedback we might get from others. This is actually a tried-and-true part of a typical assessment for drug addiction problems, as respondents get asked whether, or not, other people have suggested that the respondent has a problem. The idea here isn't, in any case, self-indictment. There's nothing "bad" about being overcharged, or defensive, or emotionally cool. These are all just traits that tell us something about how we manage our energy, not about whether, or not, we're likable.

As for the question about pleasurable activity, think about laughter, playfulness, sensual activity, but especially about sex and orgasm. Entire books have, of course, been written about the subject and nothing stirs up more controversy. But this is a very important matter in bioenergetics and ought to be assessed honestly and without prejudice.

Reich spent virtually his entire career exploring the bioenergetic importance of the orgasm. While much criticism was directed at him for his emphasis on "orgastic potency" as the single most important criterion of mind/body health, no one has ever really suggested that the experience of orgasm is irrelevant to health and well-being. Moreover, much of the criticism that Reich endured here was based in a mis-understanding of his work. He never advocated for promiscuity, sexual exploitation of his clientele, orgasm as a treatment for cancer, or any number of other scurrilous accusations that had been made against him. And by "orgastic potency," Reich was referring to the matter of complete energetic discharge, not dissimilar to what can happen through deep belly laughter, intense sobbing, or, even, screaming in pain, fear, or anger. It is absolutely not a reference to compulsive sexual obsession or an advocacy of pornography. As a matter of fact, pornographic sex is in some ways, the opposite of fully pleasurable, orgasmic sex, as the emphasis is much more on quantity than quality. Psychologist Charles Kelly, noted neo-Reichian researcher and founder of the Radix Institute, made a most poignant statement about pornography when he pointed to its ironic similarity to moralism. The former, Dr. Kelly noted, is characterized by sex without love, the latter by love without sex. The capacity to experience deep sexual pleasure is an important indicator of bioenergetic status and may be directly linked with the capacity to experience other kinds of joy and emotional release. It needs to be considered honestly and without judgment.

After working through the questions, you should be able to find your place on the map, and a bioenergetic character type that fits. The journey to your centerpoint is now well underway.

11

Getting Unstuck

OVER 100 YEARS ago, biologist Richard Semon sought to explain how memories get stored in the brain. Semon's idea was that a trace of a new experience would get imprinted somewhere in the brain on cells "energetically predisposed to such inscription." He called those imprints engrams. While no one's yet to see an engram, the idea remains compelling.

Everything we know, believe, remember, every habit and pattern, gets encoded in the brain, somehow, whether chemically, electrically, energetically, physiologically, multi-dimensionally, or some combination thereof. So when we're talking about learning something new—creating a new memory—we're pointing to new encoding, new neural circuits, new engrams. This is important to keep in mind as we begin a journey into personal change because the old engrams don't just disappear when we make new ones. They linger. And unless we take steps to get used to thinking and behaving in a different way, the old ways will continue to get triggered and keep us stuck in old patterns. Short of surgically excising an old engram—and we've yet to even find one of the darned things—ensuring that one of our "new memories" really becomes part of who we are (and not just something we read in a book) requires that we transform what we remember, what we learn, into actual change.

What I mean by "actual change" means living life differently in both mind and body. Breaking free of old patterns and developing new ones. And summoning the will to keep practicing new ways of being over and over so the new pattern becomes stronger than the old one—stronger and more accessible.

It is one thing to believe in something. It is another thing to live like you believe in that something. If you believe it's a good idea to find greater energetic balance and get unstuck, you need to make choices in your life to reflect and support that belief. That's how you build powerful, positive new engrams. You channel your mental energy into more life-affirming, loving thoughts and authentic expression and your body's energy into greater emotional range and more graceful movement. When you bring mind and body together, you create lasting, meaningful change. Excitement, alone, doesn't create durable new neural circuits. Learning doesn't really get anchored into one's life, one's way of being-in-the-world, without practice, without consistent experiential mind/body reinforcement.

In my personal experience, acting "as if" we believe in something is a powerful tool. It's also a tool best employed consciously and with positive intent. What would happen were you to purposefully shift your breathing pattern or your posture or begin speaking more assertively or spent half an hour sitting quietly in the middle of each day? What would happen if we began to live and act like that person whom we imagine we'd be were we at our centerpoint?

Ironically, we've been engaged in this process unconsciously throughout our lives. Many, if not most, of our traits were nurtured at least as much as they were born into us. The way we hold ourselves in this world may have something to do with our genetics, but certainly has a lot to do with our life experience. We've learned everything we believe and all of the behaviors we engage in to sustain those beliefs. The durable engrams we've developed have gotten firmly etched into our brains through years and years of repetition.

Malcolm Gladwell, in his book, "Outliers," tried to explain how extraordinarily accomplished people got to be the way they are. One of the conclusions he drew is that such people spend "10,000 hours" learning, honing, perfecting their particular skill or talent. I've got no idea if that is a correct figure, but I certainly have no qualms accepting the idea that becoming great at something may require a good deal of practice.

Each one of us is already extraordinarily accomplished at being the person we've created ourselves to be. Through thousands of hours of practice, we've gotten to be where and who we are. Getting unstuck might not require thousands of hours, but it's going to require time, awareness, and diligence.

No matter where you find yourself on the bioenergetic

map, moving towards your centerpoint and getting unstuck has got to be a mind/body experience. Psychotherapy has always been limited as a vehicle for personal growth by its lack of emphasis on the body. Body-oriented methods, like Rolfing, have been limited by their lack of emphasis on the mind. We use both body and mind to manage energy and if we don't involve both body and mind in our efforts to manage our energy differently, we risk staying stuck. Without change in body and mind, the past will continue to re-assert itself. The routines of energy management we've all been using are very deeply ingrained and the ego is interested only in perpetuating what already is. Old habits die hard.

While getting unstuck may be a highly personal, individualized experience, it's an interpersonal experience, too. We are, after all, social creatures and we have developed relationships that have, like our personal thoughts and behaviors, helped to sustain our habits of energy management. Our relationships, the people that we draw into our lives, are a reflection of our relationship with ourselves and our energetic habits. Our relationships help to sustain the ways we've been managing our energy. The undercharged person will tend to seek out overcharged people with "energy to spare," and vice versa. Like the attraction of opposite magnetic poles, people seek to make connections with those who complement them energetically.

In any relationship between two people, there is an agreement, usually unspoken, about personal power, which is, really, an agreement about energy. In healthy, growing relationships, one person gives and the other receives. One teaches and the other learns. And then the roles reverse. Yin and yang. Yang and yin. In healthy, growing relationships, the agreement is flexible and evolves with the times. Unhealthy relationships get stuck on the initial agreement. If one person grows and wants something different for herself energetically—such as wanting to express feelings more freely—-the unhealthy agreement resists the change. Ultimately, one of three things will happen: the agreement will, after some struggle, get changed; or, the growing person will stop growing and revert back to form; or the relationship will fall apart. The energetic character of a relationship is, just as in the individual person, the foundation upon which the rest of the relationship is built.

What has come to be called "co-dependency" is a great example of an unhealthy relationship in which the basic energetic agreement is stuck. "Co-dependency" was originally used to describe an alcoholic relationship in which one person was alcohol-dependent and the other (the "co-dependent") enabled the addiction. But, more recently, the term has taken on a much broader meaning. Now, "co-dependent" is used to describe anyone in a relationship in which a partner's needs and feelings matter more than one's own, so there are, typically, a lot of efforts made to keep the "other" happy, even if it means denying, or hurting, one's self. "Co-dependency" has also been described as "relationship addiction," inasmuch as the co-dependent person holds on to a relationship, just as a person might continue to abuse alcohol, even though the relationship is costing them their well-being.

Whatever term you might use, the core feature of this kind of relationship is that it is stuck in a destructive, life-negative pattern where there's no personal growth.

In the process of getting unstuck from our old energetic patterns, the agreements we've made in our relationships are going to get challenged. Such challenges can mean some hurt feelings and disappointments. It is not only we, ourselves, that have gotten used to our energetic patterns. The people in our lives have gotten used to them, too. This is even more the case with the people we're closest to, and that would include our friends, family, partners, and spouses. The ways in which we've managed our energy have been part of the agreements we've made in these relationships and, if the relationship can't endure a shift in the agreement, one's personal growth is going to be perceived as a threat.

It might seem strange to think that, in the context of what has seemed a loving relationship, one's personal growth might be perceived as threatening, but that's often the reality. People who, for example, fall in love at age 25, fall in love with that other person at that time. They fall in love with the person who manages her energy in that particular way. In a healthy relationship, in which both parties continue to grow, love flourishes, as the initial agreement(s) the two people made evolve over time with the new experience and learning that accumulates. But, in an unhealthy relationship such as what gets called "co-dependent," the fear of change can overwhelm the love of life and growth. The fear of angering, or disappointing, one's partner can be paralyzing. Such paralysis is antithetical to the business of getting unstuck.

Just as it might seem strange to think that a loving relationship might be threatened by personal growth, the idea that the agreements we make in our relationships shouldn't be subject to change ought to seem downright bizarre. Who, after all, would even want to be the same person at 40 that they were at 25? Aren't change and growth amongst the hallmarks of a life well-lived? Why would anyone who values their life want to be in a relationship, in a partnership or marriage, in which agreements aren't subject to revision—especially when those revisions are all about greater health, vitality, self-esteem, pleasure, and balance?

It bears repeating that the most loving thing one can do for another person is to love them, which means, among other things, that you don't fear them. If getting unstuck means that I have to express my angry feelings more directly, then the most loving thing I can do for myself—and for my partner—-is to express my angry feelings more directly. If my intention is to get unstuck, then my partner's discomfort or disappointment can't be helped. It's just something my partner has to deal with. It's grist for his mill, so to speak.

If getting unstuck means expressing my angry feelings more directly and I don't do it out of fear, I not only keep myself stuck in an unhealthy energetic pattern. I enable my partner to stay stuck, as well. Hint: that's not love.

Focusing now on the bioenergetic map, there are, basically,

four types of energetic characters referred to simply as I,II, III, and IV. Each type represents a distinct mind/body pattern of energy management. Those patterns are each characterized by certain trends in mind/body behavior which include ways of carrying one's self in the world and dealing with one's emotions. Within each type, there is a virtually unlimited number of subtypes, distinguished by the pre-eminence or intensity of any single trait, or group of traits. Movement towards the centerpoint is easy to envision on the map as movement towards the other pole of the bioenergetic axis. To move towards his/her centerpoint, the underbounded must explore becoming more bounded; the overbounded must explore becoming less bounded, and so forth.

Type I

Type I people tend towards an overbounded mind and an underbounded body. The overboundedness in the mind tends to compensate for the underboundedness in the body. This is how a functional energetic balance gets maintained. The overbounded mind is a defensive mind, which means, basically, that this person uses his thoughts and words to defend his personal space. He has to use his mind in this way, because his body tends towards openness and vulnerability. In other words, this is someone who feels things deeply but uses his mind to keep things under control. He's energetically "open" in body but "closed" in mind. He likely trusts his mind, more than his body, to keep him safe. The more shame and trauma to which he's been subject in his life —-this is true for all

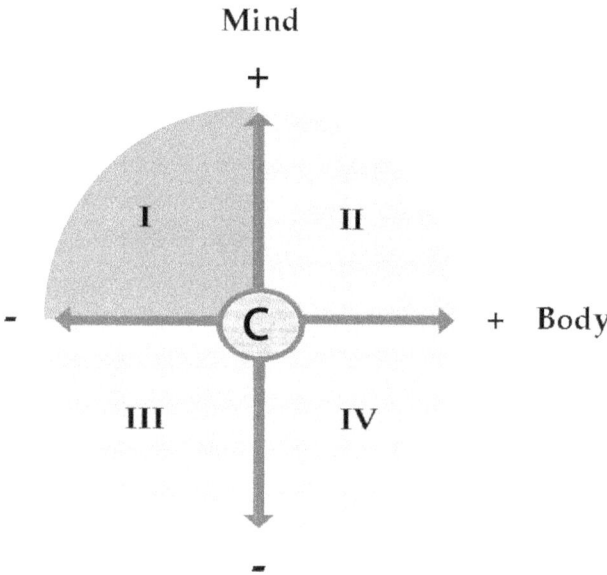

Types—-the farther from his centerpoint he finds himself on the bioenergetic map. Getting unstuck for this person means developing more physical armoring and letting go of some of the mental armor—-learning to contain his physical energy better and, as he does that, being less psychologically defensive. The one will help enable the other.

Psychological defensiveness can take many forms. Freud, of course, wrote extensively on the subject and included in his descriptions of "defense mechanisms" not only those behaviors people use to protect their personal space from others, but those they use to hide the truth from themselves, as well. Concepts like "denial" and "projection" and "repression" are pretty well universally understood. People defend themselves from what they perceive to be threats from "out there" but they also try to protect themselves from threats from within. We may be disturbed by what others might say or do, but we might also be disturbed by memories and feelings we already have.

Becoming less psychologically defensive means, basically, to stop pushing out at the world and stop fighting with reality. Be more yielding and welcoming. Listen more than you speak. Be inquisitive rather than dismissive. Some mental defensiveness may be necessary to help protect one's personal space, but too much results in mental isolation: no one can get close to the person who never lets anyone in.

The single most salient characteristic of the psychologically defensive person is "No."

That's his (or her) response to new information, new ideas, new sensations, new realities, new possibilities. The defensive person is, by definition, well-protected, but also lonely and stagnant. You can't get close to anybody or learn anything new when your most common response to new experience is "No." You can't get unstuck when you insist on remaining right where you are.

To move towards his centerpoint, the Type I person is going to have to start saying "Yes" more of the time. "Yes" to other people's feelings and ideas and "Yes" to his own inner life. He (or she) will need to practice over and over again being more welcoming and receptive. As fears of getting enmeshed might surface, he's going to need to confront those fears realistically, in part by asking whether, or not, he really has cause to be afraid. Is this other person really out to control him? Is this other person really unsafe? Should I continue to deny my real feelings or should I listen to them more? Does it really make sense for me to cling to this old idea that, "unless I defend myself, my identity will be destroyed?" That's half the work. The other half has to do with his body.

The underbounded body allows for energy to move too freely so that the person feels too much. People with underbounded bodies are capable of deep physical and emotional intimacy but have a tough time containing their energy when they need to. This can render them undercharged and dependent on others for energy. It can also render them more vulnerable and prone to impulsivity.

Underboundedness shows up in the body as a relative lack of muscular development (softness) through the upper torso, consistent with a relative shallowness in breathing and a less secure bearing.

To get unstuck, the Type I person will need to explore the opposite side of the Body axis. In other words, he's going to need to cultivate a greater capacity to contain his physical energy and keep his impulses and emotions under his physical control. To do this, he's going to have to literally develop more muscular armoring through his upper torso. One of the great challenges in that is to do it in such a way as to maintain good connection with his emotions. He needs to learn to contain as he continues to feel. Through practice, and as he builds expertise in managing his physical energy in a new way, he'll find it easier and easier to be less psychologically defensive, which will, together, set him (or her) on a solid path of personal growth.

Type II

For the Type II person, the energetic realities are different. This is a person who has an overbounded mind and an overbounded body. This is a person of very high energy and very high tension. Controlled but looking ready to explode at any moment, a Type II person manages his excessive energy by the sheer force of his physical armoring and psychological

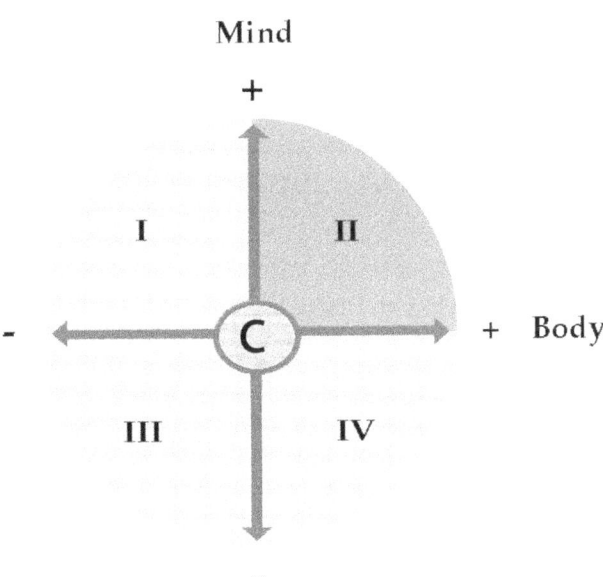

defensiveness. He is intense and can, if he loses control (which inevitably happens sometimes) be abusive to others, at least insofar as energetic explosions can feel overwhelming to people.

The main bioenergetic task for the Type II person is to soften, to allow himself to feel and receive. While a Type II person may appear to be angry much of the time, owing to his overall tension and high energy, this doesn't mean that he's necessarily ungenerous or unkind. What it means, more than anything, is that his boundaries were disrespected, if not violated, during childhood resulting in his having a distrust-ful attitude towards life. This would apply to both the world "out there" and the world within himself. Type II people are no more welcoming of their own emotions than they are the feelings of others. The energetically impenetrable appearance of the Type II person is a result of his efforts to resist feeling, not a sign of self-assuredness. If the Type II person were not "afraid to let go" and let himself feel or allow for others to get close to him, he'd never have developed so much armor in the first place. Type II people and those who work with them really need to be mindful that the fearfulness that underlies their sturdy armor is worthy of compassion, not scorn, because it is only by bringing a compassionate, loving attitude towards getting unstuck that the Type II person will be willing to soften.

The softening process for the Type II person needs to in-volve both a letting go of the tough, aggressive psychological defenses (the "No") and a loosening of the musculature to allow for more energetic flexibility. That is what movement towards the centerpoint is going to require: getting quiet and becoming a better listener, looking within for answers rather than blaming others, exhaling more freely, especially at moments of tender emotion, and learning to relax. Such softening can be challenging for a strongly Type II person (read: a Type II person who had likely been subject to significant abuse as a child) and typically requires a lot of cathartic work.

Karl, for example, was a policeman who'd come to see me after he'd been referred to his commanding officer for an "anger management problem." Karl had been accused, apparently for good reason, of assaulting a younger trainee. Because of an otherwise exemplary record, he'd been given the option of pursuing psychological treatment rather than enduring a more serious disciplinary action. Karl was in his mid-thirties, married with a young child, and had recently won a physical fitness competition in his age group. He was classically "fit," with broad shoulders, a narrowed waist with "washboard abs," a square jaw, piercing eyes, and a tough demeanor. Fortunately, he'd been humbled –at least somewhat—by his recent troubles and he brought to therapy a real willingness to "get to the bottom" of his anger problems. But, he had virtually no insight and showed a real tendency, in speaking about the recent incident, to blame others. The young trainee was "a pussy" and his Chief was "an asshole." Karl had "never thought much" about why he had such an explosive temper, but he did recognize that he might have a problem, as he'd been in numerous fights over the course of his life with "people who think they can get away with stuff."

My first therapeutic task with Karl was to establish enough of a trusting relationship with him that he felt safe talking about his painful personal history. In fact, he'd been repeatedly physically abused by his father, who'd also been physically abusive to Karl's mother. There had been a great deal of unreported, unresolved family violence. Karl had "learned to be tough." His mother, who'd been, apparently, chronically depressed and who had died at a young age from cancer, had repeatedly turned to Karl for emotional support, even to the point of discouraging his relationship with his first girlfriend and repeatedly making extraordinary demands that he spend time with her and "be the one man in (her) life (she) could really count on." Karl used the word "oppressive" over and over again to describe his mother.

My second task with Karl was to help him understand how he coped with all the violence and violations of his personal space.

Once he began to develop that insight, I introduced him to the idea of getting unstuck, which would require, I told him, that he learn to manage his feelings differently and experiment with "not being so tough all of the time." To my pleasant surprise, Karl was willing to do that work. "Whatever it takes, Doc," I remember him saying.

That "not being so tough all the time" took a lot of work, some of which was downright messy. A heavily armored, heavily muscled person has, typically, been holding back a lot of emotion for a long period of time. His diaphragm, especially, is tight, which gets in the way of emotions flowing. When the armor starts to loosen and the diaphragm starts to swing more freely, that pent-up emotion can come roaring out. When that happened with Karl, he vomited profusely.

Yes, there were tears and vomit *au go go*.

Fortunately, I was able to grab a towel just in time. And I was grateful that Karl offered to take the soiled towel home with him to wash it. He was grateful for the emotional release and for the softening that happened in its wake. For the first time "in years," Karl said, he felt "kind of peaceful." He had touched his centerpoint and was on his way to breaking old energetic patterns for all time.

His eyes softened. His chest loosened as his exhalation deepened. He smiled and seemed receptive. He looked, for that moment, at least, like a new man. There was still a lot of work, and practice. to do, but Karl's journey towards a different way of being-in-the-world, and to getting unstuck, had begun.

Type III

If the Type II person can seem highly energized, aggressive, even domineering, the Type III person is his energetic opposite. Highly sensitive, often highly intuitive, generally withheld, usually compliant, the Type III person moves through life underbounded and undercharged. Lacking filters, the Type III person is, if anything, too open to new experience, so she's prone to making deep connections without sufficient discernment, especially if the person with whom she connects is

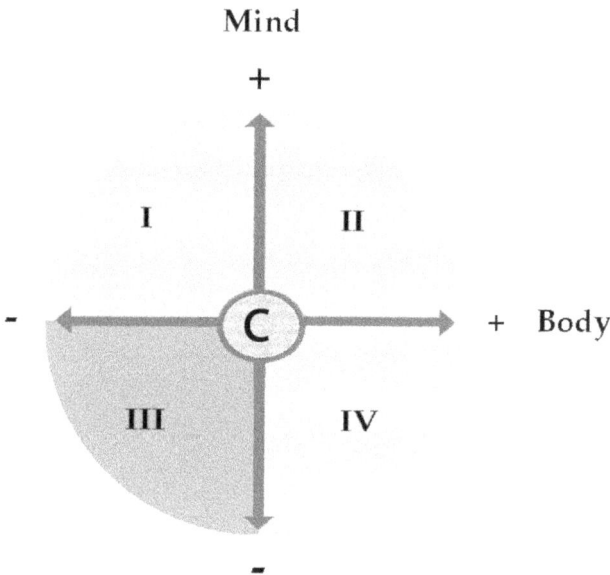

Mind

+

I   II

-    C   +   Body

III   IV

-

offering her the energy and protection she's unable to create for herself. While "letting go," in one way, or another, needs to be part of the process to get unstuck for all the other types, the Type III person's journey must involve a lot of "learning to hold it together."

It might seem strange to think that there are people for whom the building up of armor is key to their personal growth, but that's the reality for the Type III person. Armor does create barriers, but without such barriers, life would be chaotic. We all need to be able to feel fully, but also to set aside feelings when we've got work to do. Too much feeling too much of the time is a prescription for disorganization, impulsivity, drama, and crisis. Without sufficient armoring, a person can struggle to focus and complete tasks, rely too much on the energy of others, and lose a sense of his personal space. Mostly, though, the underboundedness of the Type III person results in the person feeling disempowered.

If there's any single word you might fairly use to describe the existential experience of the Type III person, that's it: disempowered. Energy doesn't get held or channeled by the Type III person. It moves through her like water through a sieve.

For the Type III person, moving towards the centerpoint means building armor both mentally and physically. Put simply, she (or he) needs to learn to hold energy in and to keep it out. This usually requires a contemporaneous building up of the musculature (in the upper body, especially) and the psychological defenses. The Type III person needs to learn how to say "No" effectively, appropriately, and in the service of getting unstuck.

Karen was in her early forties and newly divorced for the third time. She'd recently begun a new relationship with a man she'd met at a party. She'd been having panic attacks for "no reason." She was tall and thin, very pretty, but also had obviously had a lot of cosmetic surgery. She was dressed provocatively, in a short skirt, low-cut blouse, and heels. She was very open and friendly, to the point of being seductive. She was also very intelligent and articulate.

When I asked her about her personal history, Karen began almost immediately to launch into a detailed accounting of her sex life which, she claimed, started with getting molested by her mother's boyfriend when Karen was just seven years old. After a few moments, I interrupted her and asked her how she felt about sharing such intimate details of her life with a man she'd just met.

"Well, that's what I'm supposed to do, isn't it?, she replied. I said, "No, not really. What I'd like for you to do is to find out first if I'm someone you feel comfortable sharing your story with." Karen was nonplussed. "How do I do that?," she asked. "I wouldn't know where to begin." I suggested to her that she think, for a moment, about how she ever knows when it's safe for her to reveal herself to another person. After drawing a blank, Karen calmly said, "I think this is something I might need to work on. I've got a lot of regrets about men I've gotten close to. I guess my pattern has been to move into things a little too quickly..."

Karen was able to understand how her panic attacks were triggered by her fears of "losing herself" and that this seemed to come up every time she started a new romantic relationship. She was quick to grasp the idea that, if she were going to bring an end to her panic attacks, she was going to have to learn to be more discerning and make more empowered choices about her personal space. Karen felt excited by the insight and was enthusiastic about continuing in therapy.

As we finished this first session, Karen got up to leave. Upon doing so, she went to give me a hug. "Let's wait on that,

Karen," I said, "until you've learned more about your bound-aries." She stopped herself. "Right, Dr. Steve. I'll see you next week."

The work of helping Karen get unstuck from old patterns had begun, but there would prove to be a great deal more work to do. After a number of visits in which we explored matters of trust and boundaries, we moved into more of a "body-orient-ed" modality and I worked with her to open up her breathing, build more strength in her upper body (which she supple-mented with weight-lifting) and improve her grounding. I led her through exercises that would push her to tolerate more and more energetic charge without giving in to the feelings. I gave her assignments to practice assertiveness. There were some "shameful" sexual memories that had to be confronted along the way. Over and over, I gave her the message that she was worthy of being loved and respected for the person she is and recommended that, every week, at least, she do one thing to affirm that message. Along the way, the panicking stopped. Karen began to carry herself with greater assurance. She said she felt "more exuberant." I saw her getting unstuck, and it was a beautiful thing to see.

Type IV

Type IV people are physically overbounded but psychologi-cally underbounded. It is an interesting energetic equation, as Type IV people need to open up to their own needs and feel-ings while learning not to let the needs and feelings of others overwhelm them. Bioenergetic growth for the Type IV person

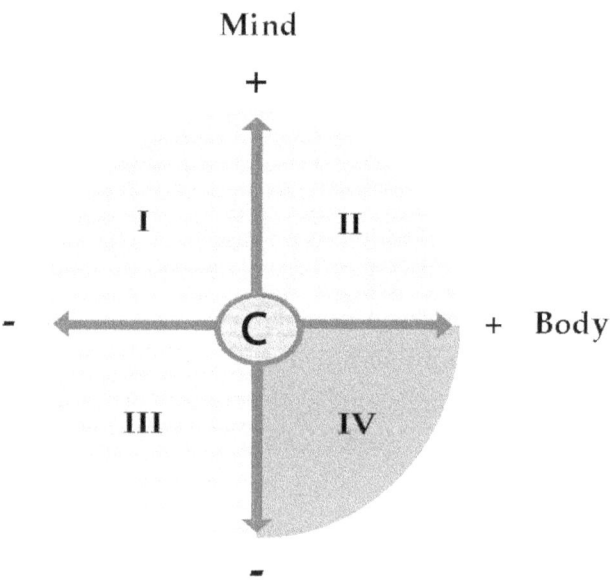

is about opening up to the flow of energy in the body while building better defenses against the energy of others.

I don't believe that "everybody wants to rule the world," but I do believe that everybody wants to feel like he's in control of his (or her) personal space. To feel in control, to feel empowered, a person's got to feel a sense of energetic balance and vigor. He's also got to have a sense of integrity about himself: that he means what he says, is who he is, and that there's a consistency to his character. Each one of us wants to feel as if our beliefs are our own, our identity is unique, our body is ours to do with as we please, and our personal space (however we define it) is ours, and ours alone. No one wants to feel like he's at the mercy of someone else's interests, feelings, or desires. No one wants to feel disempowered. This is why psychological defenses are so important. And it helps to explain why the person with inadequate psychological defenses —- the psychologically underbounded person—-might struggle so much with anxiety. The world becomes a scary place when you don't really feel you can defend yourself when you need to. Nothing, in fact, feels more disempowering than that.

The more psychologically disempowered a person feels, the more they'll try take control in their bodies. Type III people struggle with both their body armor and their psychological defenses, so their inner lives tend to be chaotic, marked by too much unchanneled, uncontained energy. The Type IV, possessed of more significant muscular armoring, can keep his inner life from being too chaotic, but he does so at the cost of a great deal of tension.

Peter was a 37 year-old dentist, married with no children. He was short in stature, but quite muscular. He had the body of a wrestler, or a gymnast, very fit and tight and energetic. He was also impeccably well-groomed. He wore glasses for near-sightedness and seemed like someone who took great pride in his appearance. He had a slightly effeminate quality about him or, at least, that was my experience. Peter had been referred to me by his primary care physician, who thought that his sudden spike in hypertension might have been "stress- related."

"Yes, sir," Peter acknowledged. "I have been under a lot of stress, lately. Dr. M said I might be able to learn some stress management techniques from you." We went on to discuss the recent "stress," with Peter all the while being polite and cooperative to the point of obsequiousness.

The "stress" Peter was referring to was that he'd recently discovered his wife had rung up $86,000 in credit card bills. Apparently, she'd become addicted to one of the "home shopping" television channels and had been "buying all kinds of stuff," then hiding the monthly invoices. A certified letter demanding payment is what had gotten Peter's attention. Peter claimed that he'd known nothing about the purchases because his wife had been secretly stashing all the merchandise at her brother's house.

"She doesn't care about anything I say, anyway," Peter said about his wife. "She's done things like this before, just not to this extent."

When I asked him how he'd dealt with it in the past, Peter sheepishly shrugged his shoulders. When I asked him how he felt about it now, he said, "I'm very upset, of course, but what can I do?"

"You could tell your wife that you're very angry and fed up and demand that she get some professional help for her compulsive spending and lying," I replied. But Peter just looked back at me, his sad eyes blank.

Getting to know Peter better over the next several weeks, I learned that, while he'd always taken a lot of pride in his appearance—he'd been working out regularly since high school and "still weighed the same as (he) did at age 21"—-he also always felt a lot of shame about all the times he'd been "a schmuck." He'd loaned money to friends on several occasions that never got repaid. Worst of all, in his mind, was he'd agreed to a three-way sexual encounter with his wife and another man, about which he could only say, "Do you know how humiliating that was?"

Peter was clearly someone who, despite his powerful capacity to maintain emotional control, felt disempowered by his inability to say "No" or express his angry feelings, a dilemma which illustrates well the energetic challenge faced by the Type IV person.

Yes, Peter needed to learn how to "manage stress" better. But, if he was going to stop re-creating the same stress-inducing scenarios over and over in his life, he was going to have to learn not just how to manage stress but also to manage his energy differently. He was going to have to allow his body to soften so that he'd be able to feel more fully and get out of denial about the emotional realities of his life. He was going to have to learn to say "No" to others while saying "Yes" to himself. He was going to have to seek empowerment and stop allowing others to disempower him. That's what it was going to take to help him get unstuck—and reduce his stress.

Would Peter's marriage be able to survive an energetic shift in Peter? Who knows? That is one of the risks in getting unstuck. The relationships we've formed and the agreements we've made while stuck might not make sense at the centerpoint. A more fully empowered, better energetically balanced, better well-defended Peter wouldn't ever be "a schmuck" again. Maybe his wife was happy with the old compliant, self-denying, too-tolerant Peter.

This is, again, where it is important to remember about choosing love rather than fear. Love is about wanting what is best for ourselves and those around us—and realizing that they're the same thing. The best thing for ourselves is what's best for those around us. If my marriage, or my friendship, or my partnership had been founded upon my being stuck, or my being disempowered, or, more simply, on my being somewhat less alive or engaged or evolved energetically than I am today, that doesn't mean that, to get unstuck, I have to end the relationship. But it does mean that the relationship is going to need to change, to evolve, to adjust, to grow. Getting unstuck may challenge a relationship, but it actually presents a wonderful opportunity for both people to learn, grow, and find greater peace together and within themselves.

12

The End of the Beginning

IT'S BEEN SAID that each of us sings a song of our life. The words change from verse to verse as we move through the ever-shifting circumstances of our lives, but the melody tends to stay the same. The choices we make and the other people we attract into our lives respond to that melody, either harmonizing with it, or providing counterpoint. It is that melody which has attracted them to us and us to them. It is that melody which is most deeply ingrained and easiest to sing. If you want to change your life and get unstuck, you need to change the melody. You need to start singing a different tune.

To sing a different tune, we've got to get unhooked from the old one. The old tune may be catchy. Lord knows it's familiar, so much so that we can sing it in our sleep. In fact, we do sing it in our sleep. We sing it all the time. Maybe singing that old tune really did help us survive a violent, unstable mother or an absent father or some other horrible trauma. So we ought to be grateful for that old tune. It helped to get us through.

But, if we keep singing that same tune, we remain, essentially, that kid who's struggling to survive. Rather than becoming an expansive, enlightened, more fully realized, more peaceful, loving person and singing a tune which reflects that reality, we stay stuck in the past. And we wind up attracting into our lives other singers who know that tune as well as we do. Change the tune and we'll change our lives. Change just the lyrics and our lives remain the same.

Substance abuse experts say that the point at which addiction begins is the point at which a person's emotional development stops. I think there is a parallel truth about being stuck: The point at which you get bio-energetically stuck in your life is when your personal growth stops.

People engage in all kinds of things to help themselves heal, help themselves get unstuck. We take drugs. We go to see shamans, gurus, re-birthers and re-programmers. We go to churches, mosques, temples, ashrams, and synagogues. We attend weekend seminars, meditate, explore our past lives and our inner child. We visit sacred sites, go gluten-free, drink less of this and more of that, fast, cleanse, and, of course, we read books like this one. We do all kinds of things to try to free ourselves from old patterns, mend our hearts, mend our bodies, and re-vitalize our lives. Healing and personal growth are not just passing fads or esoteric interests. We all want to feel as good and as free as we possibly can. We all want to be unstuck.

Back in the 1980s, I found myself horribly stuck. Though I was living in Hawaii, married to a lovely woman with two beautiful little daughters, had good work to do, and good health, I'd become miserable. I wasn't getting enough sleep. I was eating too much. The glass of wine with dinner had turned into two or three glasses. I was sullen and irritable. I had so much but was deriving no pleasure from any of it. I was depressed.

It wasn't my first bout with depression. I'd been through some bleak periods prior to this. Never suicidal, but definitely down. I am genetically pre-disposed to depression. I once went to a party and spent half the evening alone in a large upstairs closet. I was not unfamiliar with dark nights of the soul. But this time was different. This time I had other people to care for, who were dependent on me, who really noticed my absence. This time, the depression had lingered and I couldn't see a way out.

To help support my young family, I'd taken a position as clinical psychologist at a new private psychiatric hospital. I'd been friends with the medical director, who had recruited me for the job, and the lucrative salary had its allure. I went into it with excitement and great expectation. For the first year, or so, it was great. I'd become director of one of the hospital's treatment programs, which was a proverbial feather in the cap. I was making a lot money. I was getting along well with the other doctors and staff. The hospital was a lively, growing place, and I was coming home every night with interesting stories to tell.

But then, things quickly started to change.

The hospital started denying me the resources they'd promised to provide to the treatment program, so we really weren't providing the services we were advertising. That certainly didn't sit well with me. More importantly, the hospital had started morphing into what I'd been promised it wouldn't become: another dreary, profit-driven, corner-cutting, creativity-averse psychiatric holding facility. It was as if all the bright, enthusiastic energy most of us had brought into this "place to blossom and shine" (their description, not mine), had started to get vacuumed up by some monstrous corporate suction-machine. Just the kind of place I'd sworn never to be a part of.

Nevertheless, the money was good and helped to keep me narcotized, so I kept on. I was regularly putting in 45-50 hours a week at the hospital, then doing another 10-12 hours per week of private practice. I was busy, busy, busy. My bank account was growing. But my spirits were starting to sink. I wasn't growing. I wasn't enjoying my good life. If heaven means feeling at peace in one's life, I was living in hell. The hospital wasn't the only stressor in my life at the time, but it was the most consuming—and most challenging, as it was forcing me to make a fateful choice between my integrity and my fearfulness. Do I stay true to myself or sell my soul for the sake of security?

It wasn't as if I'd completely lost touch with myself and my purpose for going into psychology. I'd wanted to help change the world. Really. I'd been inspired to go into psychology, rather than medicine, by reading Wilhelm Reich, enjoying several profound LSD trips, and the prospect of being a part of something new and revolutionary. That's why I'd gone to a very progressive graduate program, done a dissertation on Rolfing, and studied Gestalt therapy. I'd intended to remain on the cutting edge. Instead, I'd started to turn into Dr. Hack, chasing dollars, prestige, and, worst of all, sacrificing my dreams. While I put on a good public act, the reality was that I was living in fear—and feeling pretty ashamed about it.

I'd begun to live in my head and not in my heart. I had a young baby daughter but returned home from work one night to find that our au pair girl knew her better than I did. I wasn't just becoming a boring, run-of-the-mill "healthcare professional," I was becoming a lousy husband and father. I wasn't having any fun with my wife and kids, wasn't engaged in my life at home, and was often angry for no apparent reason. I'd started to turn into my own father—again violating a promise I'd made to myself years before.

Energetically, I was out of balance. My basic bioenergetic tendency to be overbounded in both mind and body had become more pronounced. Under stress, I'd reverted to an old survival pattern. This is what happens. When we go through periods of intense stress, when our sympathetic nervous system is turned on too much of the time, our basic bioenergetic tendencies get intensified. The overbounded person is going to get even more tightly wound…I always had plenty of energy to fuss and argue, but little energy for pleasure. Looking back on it, I was in a lot of pain but couldn't let myself feel it or communicate about it. Despite all the good things I had in my life, I was just flat, deadened in my body, disengaged. In hindsight, it certainly wasn't the first time I'd suffered from being stuck, but it was the worst.

Then a little miracle happened. A private client of mine was going to leave Hawaii to be nearer his family on the Mainland and, so, announced that he was going to end our sessions. That evening was to be our last meeting. By way of thanking me for my help, he announced he had a small gift for me. "I don't know," he said, "but something tells me you're going to find this stuff very interesting. And, anyway, you'll probably get more out of it than I can." He handed me several copies of an obscure publication. "The Radix Journal."

The Radix Journal detailed the clinical and experimental work of Dr. Charles Kelley, a psychologist who, starting in the late-1950s, had undertaken a study of Reich's bio-energetic therapy and laboratory research. "Chuck," as he was known to his trainees, had developed a method of bioenergetic therapy (he preferred calling it "education") derived from Reich's "orgone therapy" and the "neo Reichian" bioenergetics therapy developed by Dr. Alexander Lowen.

I found the idea of "Radix work" fascinating. I'd had no idea that anyone on the planet was still doing that kind of therapy. More important to me, The Radix Institute was offering a training program. Literally, within a few days of receiving those journals, I was tracking down names and telephone numbers. A voice inside of me had said "Yes." I knew, I just knew, that this was what I needed to do to get back to myself, back to my joy, back to my passion. The only thing that would get in my way would be my job at the hospital. Could I let that go? Could

I walk away from the money and security to step back into a more radical cutting edge career?

Could I make this decision in love rather than in fear?

After a few days away from the hospital, I went back to work. I had a casual lunch with my friend, the medical director, with whom I'd shared my excitement. I might've told a few other people, as well, that I'd discovered there was this training program called "the Radix training" that I was thinking about doing. I'd just been struggling a bit with when I'd take the time off to fly to Dallas for the first seminar.

Late in the day, as I was starting to walk towards the parking lot, Michael, a psychiatrist with whom I'd worked closely and become friendly, hurried towards me with a slight look of panic on his face. "I heard that you're thinking about going to Texas to learn how to use a Rolodex. Is that really true? Are you OK?" At that moment, my decision to resign from the hospital and pursue the Radix training became crystal clear. The hospital was not me, was not my life. I had to leave there to return to myself.

Within a week, I'd made my plans and submitted my resignation. Even if the training proved a bust, I was done with the hospital, with that life, done with the compromises, the lifelessness, the pretense. I wanted to get unstuck, and returning to the kind of deep, transformative mind-body personal growth work that I'd abandoned seemed like a key to both my personal healing and my professional rebirth.

In fact, the training was anything but a bust. It was a revelation. My first time in Texas, I found myself disoriented and somewhat awed by the sheer size of everything—the houses, the ranches, the pecan groves, the monte cristo sandwiches. It was a far cry from Hawaii. But when I stepped into the conference room where the training was to be held and I saw the lively open faces of the dozen, or so, other people in the room, I felt a sense of peace. These were my people. And when the intense bioenergetic emotional release work that is Radix got underway, my excitement overwhelmed my fear. I was home. My body began to let go even before my "intensive" began. Over and over again, I found myself deeply moved by the powerful tears and screams of the other participants as they went through their individual sessions and let go of fear, pain, and anger that they'd kept locked up in their bodies. Feeling so connected with, and being privy to, such intimate emotional purges is truly a sacred experience. During my own first intensive, I kicked and hollered and felt as if I'd thrown a twenty-pound weight off my shoulders. And over the next two and a half years of personal therapy and training, I learned about just how much pent-up anger and pain a person can contain— and how liberating it feels to let it go. The experience helped me to get unstuck then and has helped to keep me on a path of personal growth ever since. I've learned to soften. I've learned to let in. I've learned to cry. I've learned not to betray myself.

The Radix work isn't for everyone. I needed a heavily body-oriented therapy that would help get me back in touch with my tender emotions and loosen up the tensions that were keeping me stuck. And I was really interested in exploring the grand energetic promises of Reich's work and bringing it into my professional practice. That's not for everyone, either.

But what may well be true for everyone looking to get unstuck is that the work, whatever form(s) it should take—bioenergetic therapy like Radix or Lowen's bioenergetics or orgonomic treatment or Rolfing or meditation or Gestalt therapy or yoga or Jungian dream interpretation or patterning or mindfulness or dialectical behavior therapy or eye movement desensitization or tantric massage or ayahuasca or prayer or making music or making love or some combination of those elements—is going to take some time. No one gets stuck overnight or gets unstuck over a weekend. A moment of great insight or when a solution to a nagging problem gets revealed is a wondrous and important event. But it's often just the end of the beginning of one's journey into greater joy and freedom. Personal growth has no goal other than greater and greater expansion of mind/body consciousness. The work is never really done.

Nor does the journey proceed in a straight line. Unstuck doesn't mean you never have to face your inner demons again or that you can completely undo or remake your genetic endowments. As much as I'd like to believe otherwise, I'll likely always have a tendency under stress to tighten in my mind and body and hold in my pain. As an unstuck person, though, I'll recognize the tensions more quickly, be honest about what I need to do to release them or transform the stuck energy into creative, purposeful behavior, and keep getting better and better at doing so. I know that, if I do that, I'll stay unstuck, even if I have a few moments of stasis along the way.

As for psychology, I hope that it can re-discover its humanistic soul. All of the "evidence-based" treatments that have been developed for anxiety and post-traumatic stress and borderline personality disorder and a whole host of other psychological illnesses are beautiful things. Many people are living better lives as a result. But there is so much more profound work that can be done.

Once, in the midst of a Radix workshop I was conducting, one of the participants—he happened to be a veteran of numerous Radix workshops as well as years of addiction recovery—blurted out, "You know, if you do this work, it changes you."

Change has always been my goal. It is the natural state of being. Even in stillness, there is change. There is movement. We breathe in and we breathe out. The heart beats. Change is fundamental to life. Stasis is not. One day is not meant to be just like the one that came before it.

As I write these last few pages, there is great strife and suffering in the world. Violence. Lack. Fear. Despair. These are all happening at a global level. But, like all events, all circumstances, all crises, they are a reflection of the consciousness of the people involved. Those worst elements of societies are also within each one of us. Our lives are, at least in part, a reflection of how we manage our energy and the thoughts and behaviors we generate. If I'm not being treated well that is, somehow, a reflection of my own negativity. If a group is not being treated well, that is, somehow, too, a reflection of the negativity of the group—even if that negativity is just a matter of silent, unspoken prejudices, fears, hatreds, and recriminations.

As I looked back on my experience at the hospital, I realize that such places, too, are a reflection of the energies that the people who work at such places bring to the job. Perhaps I am wrong, but I think the "stuck" atmosphere of the hospital had been a reflection of the collective stuck energy of the administrators, the doctors, and the nurses. We'd created it and not the other way around.

Personal growth is a powerful force. It really is no wonder that it might meet up with resistance from both within us and around us. We don't know where, exactly, or to what, it's going to lead. We can understand that the centerpoint is a place of energetic balance inside us, but we don't know what a life lived closer to that centerpoint is going to look like. The more strongly we cling to the way things have been or the way we think they ought to be, the more resistant we are to change. Even in our suffering, we cling to what's familiar because the familiar is what we trust.

With growth and change comes uncertainty, and it is a peculiar characteristic of humans that we'll choose what we know already over what we don't yet know, even if what we already know has been drained of all its juice. Curiosity might be lethal for cats, but for humans, it's essential. Without it, there can be no growth.

If you fear getting unstuck because you're concerned that your current path—your relationships and/or your work— would be threatened by change or by your having a deeper, more honest relationship with yourself—I would suggest that your purpose here in this life is to live as well, and with as much love and joy, as you possibly can. You're not here to tread water. You're not here to suffer. You're not here to ensure the happiness of others. Your highest purpose is not to help co-create misery for others by discouraging their growth or by welcoming their efforts to discourage yours. When we don't express ourselves fully, we encourage others only to do the same. If I'm stuck, I encourage you to be stuck, as well. If I get unstuck, I encourage your growth as well as my own.

Of course, personal growth can be disruptive. Chaos sometimes goes with the territory. Getting unhooked from familiar patterns can leave us, at least for a moment, "betwixt and between." But without some chaos, there can be no creativity. Nothing new can come from what already is unless you shake up what already is. There are good reasons why New York City, with its seemingly endless noise and craziness, is one of the most artistically creative places in the universe while places that are more controlled, regimented, and orderly rarely are hotbeds of creativity. Genius transcends what's been given; it doesn't follow the rules. A life that allows for some chaos provides fertile ground for some new higher order to emerge.

What you might need to do to get unstuck is, in the end, up to you. You know something now about how you manage your energy. You understand what direction you need to go in to get unstuck. Hopefully, you appreciate that getting unstuck requires not just time and commitment, but also some assistance.

If you've discovered that you tend to be overbounded, you might seek out the assistance of someone who can help you loosen up, discharge pent-up emotion, reconsider your rigid boundaries, and find greater relaxation. If, on the other hand, you've discovered that you need to learn to contain your energy better, you might want to look for someone who can help you to do that. There is a wide variety of methods, practitioners, and teachers out there from which to choose. Be your own contractor. Hire the assistance you need. Use your awareness and your intelligence and your intuition.

Keep in mind that for most people, if not all, the work of getting unstuck is not easy. No matter how distressing or ill at ease we might feel our lives have become, no matter how ready, or how excited we are about healing and transformation and getting unstuck, we've gotten very, very used to those old patterns. They are as familiar to us as the sound of our own voice, more comfortable than the proverbial pair of old shoes, and the easiest song you have ever sung. It's also the thing at which you are most expert: being the person you have been.

However much education you've had, whether you've got a Ph.D. in physics or twenty-seven years repairing Swiss watches, or you've given thousands of haircuts, handshakes, kisses-on-the-cheek, or compliments, the thing you know most about, and are best at doing is being you. And that is the "you," no matter the frustrations, mistakes, and failures, who has survived, who has endured, who has gotten to this point.

Caterpillars shed their skins as they grow and change. We humans have to keep working with what we've got, with what we've been given. We've got to stretch and sometimes even "feel the burn" as we grapple with the skin of our old, stuck patterns. We can't just "shed" them. And we won't just loosen our grip on them, either, without a fight.

Oscar Ichazo, founder of the Arica school, wrote a play called "The Wall," which, quite simply, portrayed a man repeatedly striving to climb a wall, but mostly failing. He succeeds only once he realizes that the wall he's been trying to scale is not "out there," at all.

I could tell you dozens of stories of people I know, or have worked with, who felt like they'd "really gotten it" after an intensive workshop, an LSD trip, an encounter with a charismatic channeler or guru or a great, spectacular, life-changing orgasm. And then they came crashing back down to Earth. The exhilarating high of the weekend gave way to the realities of Monday morning. None of which is meant to suggest that moments of heightened clarity, extraordinary community, overwhelming pleasure, uncontrollable laughter, or mind-expanding revelation lack meaning or value. To the contrary. It's just that, in the bigger picture of our lives, such moments of *satori* provide us just a glimpse of what might be, were we to do the work it takes to get there, and remain there most of the time. Enlightenment can't be given to you; it has to be attained.

Fritz Perls once wrote "to suffer one's own death and be reborn is not easy." Buddhist teacher Jack Kornfield put it even more elegantly when he wrote "after the ecstasy, the laundry."

The truth is that personal growth is hard work and never complete. Nearly a half century of paying attention, trying to re-frame, re-work, re-call, re-wind, re-habilitate, and re-lax, and I still sometimes get triggered. The petulant kid is not gone and will never be forgotten. Not by me, in any case.

But practice need not lead to perfection to be valuable. There is great inherent value in the practice, itself. Simply bringing one's regular attention to the task of getting unstuck will make a positive difference. And if I set my sights on progress, rather than on perfection, I can find joy in the small victories and maybe even find it easier to forgive or, better yet, laugh at those times when I hit the wall, struggle, or get bogged-down in the mundanities of life.

Anyone can be a spiritual warrior.

Getting unstuck is not a matter of fixing everything that might be, or feel, wrong with one's life. While this new positive psychology strives to be more inclusive and expansive, there is much more to life than what might be understood from learning about, and working with, one's bioenergetics. Love and faith and fate and luck and miracles and mysteries and all kinds of other things make up a life and much of that is beyond what we can explain. And each of us defines "good" and "bad" and "happy" and "satisfying" and "success" in our own, marvelously idiosyncratic way. You buys yer ticket and you takes yer chances.

This book is not meant to "crack the code." There is no code. There are a thousand codes. Will getting unstuck make you happy? I don't know. But how would it be to be happy-er? Will getting unstuck bring you peace? Maybe. But would becoming more peace-full be a good enough reason to try?

I certainly believe that becoming happier, more relaxed, feeling a greater sense of peace, ease, and possibility is worth it. And I know from my own experience, and the experiences of the hundreds of people who have been kind, and generous, and trusting, and desperate, and hungry, and brave enough to allow me to assist them in their journeys to get unstuck that it's worth it.

We've all relied on the survival skills and core beliefs we learned as young children to get through our lives. They worked. They helped to get us through. Trying to get through, or, better yet, trying to thrive with a different set of skills and beliefs might seem scary, daunting, maybe even impossible.

But what you have already done, what you've already survived, might very well seem scary, daunting, or impossible to someone else. The multi-dimensionality of human life and consciousness creates a vast, vast field of almost infinite possibility. And getting unstuck doesn't require that you erase any of what you already know. It just invites you to step into that infinite field. At your own pace. In your own way. On your own time.

Your journey into a life of greater possibility has already begun. Let this book serve not as a prescription, but as a guide to empower you to make good truthful choices out of love. You are at the end of your beginning now and the rest of your journey awaits.

May you live through interesting times.

About the Author

Dr. Steve Orenstein is a clinical psychologist who lives in Hawaii. Readers who seek more information about his workshops and other activities may reach him at DrSO123@aol.com.

Lightning Source UK Ltd.
Milton Keynes UK
UKHW041142061220
374726UK00001B/20